The Health Care Organizational Survey System

Donald N. Lombardi, Ph.D.

AHA books are published by American Hospital Publishing, Inc.,
an American Hospital Association company

Library of Congress Cataloging-in-Publication Data

Lombardi, Donald N., 1956–
    The health care organizational survey system / Donald N. Lombardi.
       p.   cm.
    ISBN 1-55648-118-7 (pbk.)
    1.   Health facilities—Employees—Attitudes—Measurement.
    2.   Employee attitude surveys.   I.   Title.
    [DNLM: 1.   Attitude of Health Personnel.   2.   Morale.   3.   Delivery
of Health Care—organization & administration—United States.
4.   Data Collection.   WX   160   L842h   1994]
    RA971.35.L653   1994
    362.1'068'3—dc20
    DNLM/DLC
    for Library of Congress   94-4528
                                              CIP

Catalog no. 088175

©1994 by American Hospital Publishing, Inc.,
an American Hospital Association company

Printed in the USA

AHA is a service mark of the American Hospital Association used under license by American Hospital Publishing, Inc.

Text set in Sabon
2.5M—5/94—0370

Richard Hill, Acquisitions/Development Editor
Anne Hermann, Production Editor
Peggy DuMais, Production Coordinator
Luke Smith, Cover Designer
Marcia Bottoms, Books Division Assistant Director
Brian Schenk, Books Division Director

To Deborah Ann

Contents

List of Figures

About the Author

Donald N. Lombardi, Ph.D., is the principal partner of CHR/InterVista, a health care human resources consulting firm headquartered in Hacketts-town, New Jersey. He has designed and implemented human resources systems in more than 150 health care organizations and conducts over 60 health care management seminars every year. He holds more than 50 U.S. copyrights on health care management systems and is the author of numerous books and articles, several of which are considered the definitive texts in their areas. Prior to establishing his consulting practice, Dr. Lombardi held top personnel positions at American Hospital Supply Corporation and Bristol-Myers Corporation, where he was instrumental in innovating management systems and training programs in the company's North American, Caribbean, and European operations.

As an officer in the U.S. Marine Corps, Dr. Lombardi designed several educational and manpower management programs that were lauded by both military and civilian experts. Additionally, he has designed and teaches four accreditation courses for the American College of Healthcare Executives and is a senior fellow of the Governance Institute.

Acknowledgments

This book is the result of the efforts of several other individuals in addition to myself. First, my entire family has always encouraged me in my education and professional endeavors, so all my work is a natural product of their support. The entire staff at American Hospital Publishing have again enabled me to produce a book that I believe will be helpful and progressive for the health care management community. I am particularly in the professional debt of Anne Hermann for her terrific editing and Rick Hill for his great insight and support. Daina-Lin Barbito did an outstanding job in producing the manuscript draft and assisting in the basic formulation of this book. Finally, as always, my wife Deborah Ann continues to be my most important influence and advocate. This book is just another small token of my gratitude to her.

Chapter 1 ══════════════════════════════════

System Overview and Organizational Applications

══

Introduction

Surveys have made an indelible mark on the American psyche. Most consumers in modern American society have completed some type of survey—a consumer poll conducted at a local shopping mall or a questionnaire distributed by a manufacturing company or service organization and mailed throughout a targeted area. The average American voter has become accustomed to viewing political surveys on television, and some even predicate their own voting decisions on the results of political surveys.

Likewise, most employees and managers in American business have participated in climate or attitude surveys. The surveys, which may be used interchangeably, achieve a collective sense of the opinions, input, and reactions of members of specific organizations. Attitude surveys help organizational managers set plans, take corrective actions, and gain a wide-scale sense of employee sentiment. Because surveys have become a part of regular American life, most members of organizations have an interest in the results of the survey and are more than willing to participate in the survey process by expressing candid opinions and viewpoints.

Health care attitude surveys have become prominent in the past 20 years. As health care human resources specialists have become more sophisticated and knowledgeable about their craft, they have created attitude surveys that support organizational development. When a survey is done correctly, it can produce meaningful data and valuable insights that help organizations become more innovative. However, when done incorrectly, attitude surveys may foster disharmony and mistrust and close down communications; that is, they may unintentionally defeat the very purpose for which they were constructed.

In this chapter, an overview of the benefits and liabilities of a health care attitude survey system is provided and the components of a system that has been used successfully in numerous health care organizations introduced.

The objectives and benefits of a health care attitude survey, the essential components of a sound system, and the process that should be utilized in implementing such a system are also discussed.

Survey Objectives

Attitude surveys can achieve many clear-cut and attainable objectives. Most organizations initially approach the idea of conducting an attitude survey with the thought that it "would be a good idea to determine what employees are thinking." This is indeed an important goal in and of itself. It is important for a health care organization to consider an attitude survey as an essential part of its human resources strategies and ongoing employee relations efforts. An attitude survey fully and correctly utilized can achieve more broad-based objectives. The following subsections discuss some of these objectives in more detail.

Validation, Revelation, or Innovation

Most intelligent managers have a good idea of the attitudes of employees and the overall climate of the organization. At its most basic, an attitude survey used correctly can validate the accuracy of management's perceptions of the organization. Also, the attitude survey can help management more specifically address workplace deficiencies and concerns, as well as capitalize and build on acknowledged program and personnel strengths.

Attitude surveys can also reveal certain trends within the organization. For example, there may be some previously undetected employee resistance to a particular organizational objective or program. Because attitude surveys are conducted confidentially, employees usually feel more comfortable expressing their ideas freely. Often, individuals comment on specific aspects of organizational management more directly and honestly in responding to surveys than they would in participating in everyday conversations with managers. Revelations based on survey results help managers gain insight into how issues can be better addressed and projects more fully implemented.

Another important aspect of attitude surveys is that they provide a wellspring of new ideas. New ideas and innovations, of course, are crucial to the success of any health care organization, especially in situations where facilities must learn to "do more with less." Because employees are the experts at their particular jobs, it is only reasonable to solicit new ideas from them not only about their particular jobs, but also about the overall conduct of the workplace. Most employees do not perceive their organizational role as being one of an advisor to the organization. When the survey is constructed correctly and in a manner similar to the instrument contained in appendix A of this book, the responding employee has numerous opportunities to present new ideas and unique insights. New ideas cover the range of organizational action, from job content on an individual basis to overall organizational planning and strategic action. Again, because of the confidential nature of the survey, employees often are willing to provide creative solutions and innovative ideas more directly than they might in a controlled setting or in direct communication.

Morale and Motivation

An attitude survey often acts as a catalyst in upgrading morale and increasing motivation organizationwide. In a very tangible manner, each employee is given the opportunity to present his or her ideas, express his or her viewpoints, and in a sense "vote" on what type of organization he or she would like to have. When employees are provided the opportunity and encouragement to express their opinions, employee morale is bound to take a positive turn. Put simply, the attitude survey can make each employee feel as though he or she is indeed an "owner" of the business, particularly if his or her feedback and input are acted on and recognized as meaningful.

Conducting a survey is a genuine expression of management's interest in employees' attitudes; this interest reinforces each employee's sense of self-esteem and organizational affiliation. These two factors are primary motivators in any industry and are particularly strong motivating factors in health care.

Quality Improvement

With the emphasis on continuous quality improvement in health care today, it is vital to understand how attitude surveys are natural allies of the organization's quality improvement initiative. Quality begins with people. The mainstay of any quality improvement program is the participation of employees in progressive and constructive discussions about strategies to improve the organization's overall delivery of high-quality health care. Every employee can potentially contribute a wealth of information. Health care employees are extremely perceptive, particularly in relation to people and the reactions of customers (patients and visitors) in the health care setting. Employees are the experts on what is appropriate, productive, and advantageous for the organization in providing high-quality health care. Unfortunately, sometimes quality circles (groups of 10 to 12 employees discussing specific suggestions for productivity enhancement) unintentionally prohibit the participation of less talkative members of a work group. The discussions may not pinpoint a specific area of concern, or they may not allow a general consideration of all quality improvement issues.

A strong attitude survey can provide employees with the opportunity to express their perspectives on salient quality issues as well as their general opinions on other key issues. Any or all of the employees' comments or suggestions may have potential application to the organization's ongoing quality improvement efforts.

Employee and Management Development

The input provided by employees in an attitude survey—particularly that provided by technical and management employees—can be used in constructing sound development plans for the organization as well as for specific groups of employees. Employee and management development related to quality is key to the objective of maximizing an organization's performance potential. Human resource development specialists ideally begin their efforts with a needs analysis (a concerted effort to determine the specific educational and developmental needs of an individual key employee or a collective set of employees). A needs analysis often generates training and group education that, in turn, generates higher employee expertise and technical acumen.

An attitude survey can also assist the training specialist as well as the organization in determining key development areas. In such a survey, most employees make direct suggestions about the type of training they desire. However, their comments may also provide secondary, less direct information for management. For example, an employee may rate the organization as not being particularly communicative in certain areas. These comments may logically encourage the organization to make a determination to conduct management training to resolve this deficiency. Another example of "secondary information" to be acted on by management could be that a set of employees express in their survey responses that they feel as though they are not fully qualified to handle a particular responsibility. The obvious reaction to this information would be for management to provide a training session that would help employees to increase their proficiency in that particular area.

Strategic Planning

Another organizational objective that can be fulfilled by a strong attitude survey is the uncovering of information that can be incorporated into overall strategic planning. Most employees of a typical health care organization (such as a medium-sized community hospital) are also residents of the community the hospital services. Therefore, these employees can provide insight into upcoming marketing plans and community relations efforts that could be incorporated into the organization's strategic plan. Additionally, the respondents often provide a wealth of information on internal issues germane to strategic planning. For example, the organization may be planning a major, new construction project. This type of project, of course, has implications for all employees. Because management should be vitally interested in the perception and reactions of the employees to such projects, questions about such types of change should be integrated into the conduct of the survey.

To gather this type of information from employees, the survey can ask questions directly or they can be posed in the comment and suggestion section at the bottom of each page of the survey (as in the instrument reproduced in appendix A.) For example, if a new compensation program is to be implemented or specific employee relations issues need to be addressed, responding employees should be provided opportunities in the survey to express their opinions and voice suggestions.

Management of Organizational Change

Most industrial psychologists believe that three types of employees work in every organization (see figure 1-1). The first group (referred to in this book as the *superstars*) is made up of individuals who perform above expectations and, in fact, set the pace for the entire organization. Such employees are extremely competent and innovative, constantly discovering new and better ways of performing their duties. Superstars consistently perform at the highest possible level of performance. They are role models within the organization, and their participation in any organizational endeavor helps to "define the system." These individuals usually represent 15 to 20 percent of a sound organization's staff.

Figure 1-1. General Human Resources Composition of a Health Care Organization

Superstars	
	• Consistent, high level of performance
15–20 percent	• Proactive participation
	• Constant development and self-motivation
Steady Players	
	• Good credible performance
55–60 percent	• Solid reactive participation
	• Sound development and fair level of motivation
Nonplayers	
	• Lackluster, inconsistent performance
15–20 percent	• Contentiousness and negative participation
	• Regressive development and poor motivation

The second group of employees includes those who perform at a satisfactory level (henceforth referred to in this book as *steady players*). These individuals work hard for the organization but are not particularly motivated to stellar achievement. They expect fair wages, clear direction in their jobs, and as many resources as necessary to achieve their jobs' objectives. Steady players will, on occasion, rise to stellar performance in an emergency situation, but they are not particularly motivated to stand out from the crowd. Such individuals are usually the backbone of a sound organization. Steady players represent about 60 percent of the work force.

The third group of employees is made up of the *nonplayers,* nonperforming individuals who are contentious. Not strong contributors in terms of work performance or overall organizational action, these individuals usually act subversively and divisively in any organizational endeavor. They "go against the flow" at any given time. Most managers waste a good deal of time on these individuals before removing them from the organization. Unfortunately, nonplayers usually make up about 20 percent of the average health care organization's work force. Their main goal in the workplace is beating the system.

An attitude survey provides all three groups—superstars, steady players, and nonplayers—with an equal opportunity to participate and to have their say. In the day-to-day operations of a health care organization, the nonplayers often can give their working colleagues the perception that "things at this hospital are not that hot." An attitude survey can counter that negative perception and demonstrate numerically that these individuals are clearly in the minority. As seen in the percentages presented in the preceding paragraphs, the nonplayers usually represent no more than one-fifth of a health care staff. Therefore, their contentious behavior and subversive comments can be negated by a survey indication that 80 percent of the employees feel as though the organization is a good place to work, is moving in the right direction, communicates openly, and so on. Furthermore, because the survey gives all three employee groups the opportunity to have their say, there can be no employee excuses or justifications subsequent to conducting the survey regarding poor organizational attitudes revolving around communication and participation.

Monitoring of Change, Crisis, Culture, Communication, and Conflict

Because health care organizations are sociological organisms—diverse groups of people blending their talents toward the achievement of one common goal—constant monitoring of health care management's all-important C *factors* (change, crisis, culture, communication, conflict) must be undertaken. An objective of most attitude surveys (and specifically the one suggested and detailed in this book) is to assist organizational management in such monitoring.

First, *change* must be monitored and managed. Such changes include significant organizational change, changes in the type of health care being provided, and any structural or environmental change that directly affects employees.

Second, health care managers must react constructively to *crisis*. A crisis may be generated by environmental conditions (such as an economic downturn in the surrounding community) or by something occurring within the organization (such as the closing of a hospital wing due to declining patient census). In any case, the reaction to any crisis and the way it is handled should be evaluated. These evaluations, obtained through the survey process, become helpful tools in handling similar crises in the future.

For example, the author participated in a survey project conducted after a natural disaster that took place recently in a southern state. The survey indicated the grade the organization received from its employees in terms of how it responded to the natural disaster (in this case, a hurricane). More important, the results of the survey clearly indicated how the organization should proceed if such a natural disaster took place again. The information derived from the survey proved invaluable not only in monitoring employee attitudes organizationwide (assessing their fear and apprehension, for example), but also in devising and constructing new organizational plans.

Third, an attitude survey should also assist the organization in identifying the critical issues among the organization's *culture,* including whether the organization is acting cohesively or is split into various factions and disjointed segments. A well-constructed attitude survey can help determine the cultural norms of the organization. Monitoring this C factor can help management understand the tendencies of the organization and recognize its critical cultural components.

The fourth C factor is *communication*. The attitude survey itself is an exercise in constructive organizational communication. Again, every member of the organization is given the opportunity to provide suggestions and ideas that might benefit the organization, as well as to register any complaints or apprehensions they might have about the organization's conduct and performance. The attitude survey is a natural supplement to ongoing communication within the workplace and can be an invaluable resource in obtaining critical information.

Conflict is the fifth C factor in health care management. Conflict can occur on several levels and can help motivate or prohibit the accomplishment of objectives. Though stressful, it can enable growth and development, as well as foster new understanding and future alliances. Conversely, because dealing with conflict is time-consuming, addressing it adds to the time needed to achieve organizational progress, often leading to long-term feelings of distrust and apathy by employees. It is important for a health care organization to identify and monitor areas of conflict. Because, as previously mentioned, the attitude survey is a confidential instrument that provides an exclusive interchange between manager and employee, it is an ideal mechanism for revealing not only areas of conflict, but also ways that the conflict might be remedied.

Staff Participation

The use of an attitude survey can accomplish the organizational objective of staff participation. Individuals perceive that their participation was encouraged and valued by the organization when action is taken by the organization as a result of employee comments and suggestions. *All* members of the organization have been given an attitude survey to complete and thus have had an opportunity to participate in the management of the organization. If they have not participated, they have only themselves to blame.

Possible Problems and Practical Solutions in Initiating a Survey

When an organizational attitude survey is being initiated, it is essential for management to consider some of the possible problems that might arise and practical solutions for combatting them. Three potential problems and their practical solutions are discussed in the following subsections — absence of perceived need, suspicion of the survey's intent, and apathy toward the survey process.

Absence of Perceived Need

A prominent problem in the survey process can be the perception by employees and/or management that no survey is needed. Some individuals may consider the survey to be a waste of time or incapable of providing meaningful information. However, as noted earlier in the chapter, many objectives that have importance to the health care organization *can* be achieved through conducting an attitude survey.

Often, a demonstrated lack of interest in the attitude survey among managers and/or employees may be related to false expectations held on the part of a human resources specialist or senior management. It is unrealistic for the survey initiators to expect that people will be as excited about an attitude survey as they would be about a pay increase. However, it is realistic to expect that most employees are interested in getting their viewpoints across to management and that managers are interested in receiving the employee input.

Practically speaking, interest in the survey process can be generated through the planning and marketing activities the survey conductors generate.

(See chapters 2, 3, and 6 for further discussion.) Finally, most employees and managers *will* have an inherent interest in a survey, even if it is merely rooted in basic curiosity about the opinions and viewpoints of others.

Suspicion of the Survey's Intent

Many times, individuals within an organization may be suspicious of the survey's intent. In some organizations (typically those that have a strong union presence or have undergone substantial changes recently), the survey may be perceived — inaccurately — as being a tool that will be utilized to accomplish negative objectives. For example, an attitude survey may be perceived as a device through which individuals will be laid off, lose their jobs, or have their hours reduced.

In some organizations that have recently undergone negative change (for example, layoffs, downsizing, and financial setbacks), employees may have developed a sense of paranoia. Employees are fearful about the future and the organization's stability. Fear may also be generated in organizations by the nonplayers who have created the sense of paranoia through their contentious comments and subversive actions. Ironically, it is under these circumstances that an attitude survey can potentially benefit an organization the most. Practically speaking, an attitude survey can reinforce a sense of employee confidence and management investment.

Whatever management's reason for conducting a survey, clear communication is the key to success. All surveys should contain a letter from one of the organization's top managers (for example, the chief executive officer) that guarantees the confidentiality of responses and clearly explains the purpose of the survey. These directives should be reinforced by the action of managers and others involved in the survey process. The survey process itself often must be handled delicately and somewhat slowly. In the cases just discussed, management should acknowledge that negative change has taken place recently throughout the organization and stress interest in employees' responses to it. Employee participation should be elicited and encouraged from the very onset of the process. Employee participation from the beginning through the end of the project not only helps peak interest in the survey process but also reduces apprehension about the process, particularly among the large steady-player group. Employees will see the possibility of positive change or at the least that negative issues in the institution have been recognized and will be addressed.

Apathy toward the Survey Process

The worst employee reaction toward a survey is, "So what?" If employees see no definitive consequence or clear outcome of conducting a survey, the very purpose of conducting it is defeated before the process has even begun.

Presenting an Action Plan

It is vital for the CEO of an organization to pledge to present a definitive survey outcome (for example, an employee briefing session subsequent to survey completion in which results are presented and further input is encouraged, as well as a publication of the survey results for all interested parties). Moreover, it is important that the CEO promise to implement an action plan. (See chapter 4.) The promise of an action plan must be offered at the beginning of the survey process and the reality delivered at the end. Otherwise, management runs the risk of getting not only a "so what?" reaction during the survey, but also a "who cares?" afterward.

Achieving a Desirable Response Rate

Health care executives often worry about the prospect of a poor response rate to an attitude survey. Generally speaking, a response rate of 60 percent or better is considered excellent. The attitude survey that appears in appendix A of this book, when conducted in more than 20 health care organizations in the past three years, never failed to generate at least a 68 percent response rate. The reason for this good response is a simple, strong survey conduction process. The attitude survey must be presented openly and clearly by the CEO, and all members of management must help to "sell" the survey in a clear-cut, open manner. The benefits of the survey must be explained clearly to all employees. Finally, all survey process strategies must be directed to achieving confidential and comprehensive completion of the survey at all levels throughout the entire process.

It is impossible to predict a poor response rate prior to conducting the survey because human behavior is often difficult to predict. However, a poor response rate can be negated by conducting a strong, positive survey.

Certain groups within an organization may respond better to the survey than others. This outcome can sometimes be predicted by individual managers. For example, if a group consists of strong performers and well-motivated players, the assumption may be made that these individuals will generate a strong response rate. Conversely, it can be assumed that the poorly motivated nonplayers will not even complete the attitude surveys.

It is important, however, not to make any prejudgments prior to the survey. Well-motivated individuals may assume that everything is all right and therefore not feel compelled to complete the survey. On the other hand, those individuals disenchanted by the organization may fill out the survey in a block-vote fashion in order to express their displeasure in no uncertain terms. Each manager must make a concerted effort to present the survey without prejudgment to each member of his or her group and to encourage the employees to complete it. By doing so, managers can elicit a significant return rate from these particular groups.

Providing Clear, Direct Guidelines

Participant apathy can also revolve around issues regarding the format of the survey itself. Individuals may be leery of a poor return or concerned that the quality of responses may be overwhelmingly neutral or provide useless information. Following are some specific guidelines for constructing the survey and for encouraging maximum possible response:

1. *The format must be user friendly.* The survey format should be easy to understand and clear in scope and intention, and it should have a rating scale that can be easily understood and that remains consistent throughout the entire form.
2. *Questions must be pertinent.* The survey questions must have specific pertinence to an organization. If a question is not pertinent, either in reality or employee perception, it will not be responded to. An employee thinks, "This question stinks, so this whole survey stinks." Furthermore, the employee respondent may feel that the entire survey is invalid because it is not relevant to his or her particular situation. (All of the questions provided in this text are pertinent to any health care institution of any size for the next 10 years. However, specific questions should be drawn from this list as they apply to the present prevailing conditions in individual organizations. Appendix C provides supplementary survey items.)
3. *The questions must be timely.* All survey questions must be relevant to the point in time the survey is being conducted. If an important event is taking place (for example, a large construction project), a question related to this event should be included in the survey. Additionally, questions must be discounted if they do not have timely relevance to the conduct of the organization. For example, if the organization has recently downsized, a question about employee attitudes toward downsizing would not be very timely.
4. *Questions must be specific.* All survey questions must be specific in intent and clear in composition. Obviously, poorly worded questions can lead to misunderstandings that skew responses. Furthermore, questions not understood by respondents will not give survey conductors an accurate impression of the organization. As previously noted, the survey conductors do not want a respondent to make a blanket assumption that the survey is invalid or that the people conducting the survey "do not know what they are talking about" because the questions did not "make sense" the first time they were read. The use of test groups and pilot surveys are great techniques to ensure that the survey meets the standards of specificity of intent and clarity of composition.

It is essential to use questions that are open-ended in nature and encourage a certain amount of introspection by the respondents. The questions should encourage the expression of opinions and request agreement or disagreement to statements that are related to salient issues within the organization.

By utilizing participation at all levels for the survey, intelligent questions, and thoughtful survey techniques, the survey conductors can avoid potential problems, such as distrust of the survey results, noncredible information generated by the survey, or statistically or objectively meaningless responses. Sound survey construction and solid application are the keys to stellar survey conduct.

The Health Care Survey Process

Now that some general survey problems—absence of perceived need, suspicion of the survey's intent, and apathy toward the survey process—and their practical solutions have been discussed, the survey process itself needs to be addressed. A sound survey consists of five parts, or *phases of action,* that are essential to proper survey conduction. They are:

- Introduction and planning
- Calibration and preparation
- Distribution and collection
- Tabulation and analysis
- Action and feedback planning

Introduction and Planning

The first phase of the survey process is *introduction and planning.* In this phase, getting support for the survey process is essential. Most organizations begin the process at the senior management level and then try to get the complete support of the senior executive and his or her staff. Without this clear, complete support, the prospects for a successful survey are nil.

The initial phase of the process should also include establishing a consensus of individuals that includes middle and entry-level managers, department heads, and a representative group of employees who support the survey. By promoting the virtues of the survey and its importance throughout the organization, these individuals lay an organizational foundation of trust for the survey process. This core group helps facilitate the survey process from design through to completion.

Also in the introductory phase, the overall conduct of the survey should be explained to both managers and employees. First, the purpose of the survey should be discussed: why it is being conducted and how it will be implemented. Second, the desired survey outcomes should be discussed, including the desired rate of response and the expectation that all employees will participate at their own comfort levels. Third, the relevance of the survey to action plans, strategic initiatives, and other objectives should be communicated institutionwide. Fourth, the benefits gained, the objectives to be reached, and the overall contribution to organizational action and achievement should be discussed. (These benefits are discussed throughout the text.)

It is important that the introduction and planning phase should contain a schedule of events for the conduct of the survey. The schedule includes a point-by-point explanation of the survey process, including timing and deadlines. Scheduling helps to demystify the process and downplay and eliminate apprehension surrounding the survey process itself. A schedule further helps to establish all participants' expectations relative to the conduct of the survey and its final outcomes.

Calibration and Preparation

The second phase of survey conduct is *calibration and preparation*. In this phase, the actual survey instrument is constructed, refined, and readied for distribution. This process includes deciding questions' content, editing, and printing. Also, the cosmetics of the actual survey packet are almost as important as the content of the questions within. A combined committee of managers and employees will make a final determination on the look of the survey and its presentational appeal.

Certain mechanics of the survey process are also decided on in this phase. They include determining the distribution schedule, the mode of collection, and the methods by which the survey process will be communicated to staff and management. Individuals assigned distribution and collection responsibilities include line managers, human resources specialists, and any other individuals playing a significant role in the survey process.

The calibration and preparation phase serves as a final checkpoint for working the bugs out of the survey instrument. At the end of this phase, all participating survey team members should be satisfied with the question content and feel as though the instrument is as meaningful as possible. Additionally, all methods of disseminating and collecting the survey should have been explored and the most effective put into place so that the maximum possible response rate can be achieved.

Distribution and Collection

Three elements are essential to the *distribution and collection* phase. Confidentiality must be ensured and closely monitored throughout the process. Every effort should be made to ensure that all members of the organization are given a survey form and encouraged to respond. As many surveys as possible should be collected within a specific time limit.

Distribution and collection can take many forms. A forced distribution, in which individuals are asked to complete the survey form within a particular time period or at a particular event, such as an employee luncheon, may be used. Or individuals may be given the survey and asked to return it within two weeks to a preestablished collection point, such as a survey collection box in the human resources department. (These options will be discussed further in chapters 3, 4, and 6.) Regardless of what type of distribution and collection system is used, communication must be clear and confidentiality assured throughout the process. The key objective is to get *all* the forms out the same day with the support of *all* managers and supervisors.

Efforts to achieve the maximum response rate can include setting an established deadline for collection and sending out deadline reminders. Additionally, individuals may be asked to use a sign-in sheet when they return the form, making them eligible for a drawing or other event.

Tabulation and Analysis

The fourth phase of the survey process is *tabulation and analysis*. In this phase, all collected surveys are tabulated to determine specific results. From the beginning, there should be no perception of game playing with the results. In tabulating the responses, the survey conduct team is looking for both the quantitative results and related statistics indicated by the survey, as well as the qualitative results indicated by the comments and suggestions of the survey respondents. Significant trends and pockets of response are also analyzed as part of this process. (See chapter 4).

Four elements are extremely important to the analysis and tabulation process: insight, integrity, introspection, and intelligence. First, the use of *insight* provides an accurate perspective of not only the survey results and comments, but also the reasons behind them. Second, *integrity*—the honest, direct appraisal of all significant data—should be utilized in looking at the survey results. Third, *introspection* should be part of the survey analysis as the organization discovers its strengths and weaknesses. Fourth, the use of *intelligence* should be apparent in the entire conduct of the survey—particularly in the analysis and tabulation phase when survey results are being judged and accessed.

Action and Feedback Planning

The fifth phase of the survey process is *action and feedback planning*. Action and feedback planning should include timely communication of results. All information fed back to employees and managers should be provided on a timely basis. Such timeliness helps increase the trust and credibility factor of the survey. This phase should also include clear articulation of findings. The results of the survey should be published and communicated in a clear, user-friendly manner for all individuals interested in the survey results. Everyone should also have the opportunity to participate in the presentation of results and add any new ideas suggested by the survey results.

The survey should serve as a tool to gain a strong consensus on how to solve a problem, not to redefine an existing problem. The emphasis should be on solutions, not redefining problems. Finally, the survey results must be published proactively, before any negative response appears in its absence.

Conclusion

An attitude survey undertaken by a health care institution, if done correctly, can produce meaningful data and valuable insight. Broad-based objectives can be obtained that will help the institution become more innovative and give the employees a greater sense of participation in the direction of their specific work groups as well as the institution as a whole.

When the survey is initiated and throughout the process, certain problems may arise. Individuals may perceive that there is no need for a survey, they may be suspicious of its intent, or they may merely be apathetic. As this chapter discussed, survey initiators can proactively address these attitudes before they become problems.

Finally, process implementation itself is a five-step, action-oriented human resources planning strategy. By using the steps—introduction and planning, calibration and preparation, distribution and collection, tabulation and analysis, action and feedback planning—an organization can effect a progressive health care management strategy.

Chapter 2 ═══════════════════════════════

Planning and Communication

══

Introduction

Once an organization decides to conduct an attitude survey, the process of planning the survey and communicating with staff begins. The planning process incorporates the efforts of all organization members—from hourly workers to executives. After a survey has been distributed, managers and survey conductors have little, if any, control over the direction of, or reaction to, the survey; that is, once the survey is in the hands of potential respondents, nothing in it can be changed or altered. Therefore, the planning of the survey is crucial to the entire survey process. In this chapter, major planning objectives, communication responsibilities, and survey instrument construction (both in general characteristic and specific technique) are discussed.

Planning Objectives

The survey must be planned thoroughly and responsibilities assigned to all appropriate parties. Two most important aspects of the survey planning process are inviting senior managers, line managers, and staff to participate and establishing a realistic time line for survey completion.

Survey Planning Meetings

The survey planning process should include three meetings to take place at three different organizational levels. The first meeting is conducted by the chief executive officer (CEO) and his or her reporting staff. Also included in this meeting are the team of survey conductors—individuals from human resources, representatives from operations and other departments, and perhaps an outside consultant (see example in chapter 6). At this meeting, the organization's chief executives discuss the various aspects of the survey and agree on five objectives they wish to achieve by doing the survey. (These objectives can be some of those mentioned in chapter 1 or objectives related to some other organization-specific objectives.) Furthermore, this meeting is an opportunity for survey conductors to discuss probable outcomes, response rates, reactions, and so forth. The survey team also outlines the overall scheme for survey form, distribution, collection, and analysis. Also at this initial meeting, a target date is set for when the CEO will lead the briefing sessions to discuss survey results with all respondents and other members of the organization.

The second planning meeting is conducted by the survey conduct team and it is for line managers, notably those who have large numbers of employees reporting to them (for example, nursing managers with staffs greater than 40 members). Because these managers interact daily with a large number of employees, their participation is critical to the success of the survey process. They can encourage a great amount of support from staff. Additionally, they act as monitors, providing significant feedback to the survey team and helping identify trends that may affect the survey process. (Line managers' communication responsibilities and contributions will be discussed in more detail later in this chapter.)

The third meeting the survey conduct team holds is with a representative group of employees who have been chosen by management or have volunteered to participate. This group of employees, referred to as the *employee review panel,* not only should embrace their responsibilities in communicating information about the survey, but also should participate in reviewing and fine-tuning the survey instrument. (Their responsibilities will also be discussed in more detail later in this chapter.)

Time Line

These three groups—the CEO and his or her staff, the line managers, and representative employees—participate in the survey process from the initial planning stages to completion of the survey. The survey process itself should be planned according to a time line similar to the one illustrated in figure 2-1. The span of the time line should be three to four months from start to finish.

Figure 2-1. Progressive Survey Action Time Line

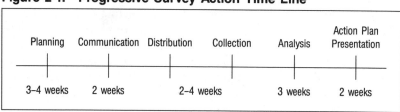

The time line indicates major checkpoints in the survey process. During planning, the instrument is reviewed and calibrated relative to the needs of the organization. Specific dates are established for communication, distribution, and so forth, and communication responsibilities are assigned. With good scheduling, the planning process usually does not take more than one month.

Two weeks should be allowed for the survey team to *presell* the survey. That is, the survey team communicates with all potential respondents regarding conduction of the survey, the survey's time frame, and the need for organizationwide employee participation. The preselling of the survey helps negate any paranoia or rumors relative to the survey's intent. However, there will always be individuals who will not believe the objectives are achievable, and no amount of preselling will convince them otherwise. However, many steady players—individuals who are relatively satisfied with the organization and their employment—will recognize that these objectives are legitimate and participate accordingly.

Optimally, the survey distribution should take two to four weeks from start to finish. This way everyone gets forms for completion at approximately the same time. Individuals should then be given two to three weeks to complete the survey. Following collection, the survey is analyzed (three weeks) and its results presented back to the organization (two weeks).

Everyone involved in the survey process—virtually the entire health care organization—should be made aware of the time line and the events that will take place relative to the survey. Communication (particularly from the outset) is critical to the entire process.

Communication Responsibilities

Communication is critical not only to planning the survey, but also to setting the correct tone for the entire process. To conduct a survey successfully, all members of the organization, but particularly the executives and managers, must be involved in the communication process. Many individuals fear that lack of leadership and a good communication network institutionwide will create and perpetuate shortcomings in the delivery of high-quality health care and job satisfaction. This fear is rooted in reality. Often, when individuals are not provided clear direction and inspiration by strong leadership, there is more opportunity for the dissatisfied employees and nonplayers to grouse. Individuals uninformed about changing organizational dynamics often spread rumors and innuendos. Therefore, clear communication by strong leaders from the outset of the survey process can help reassure all employees that the survey is *everyone's* project.

The following subsections explore executive and management communication generally and the distinctions between the responsibilities of executives and managers specifically.

General Responsibilities

As stated previously, communication by executives and managers demystifies the process and reduces feelings of ambiguity and paranoia about the survey's intents and objectives among employees. Communication can take the form of both emotional and benefit bonuses. For example, emotional encouragement includes reminding employees that they are "voting" on the future of the organization when they complete the survey. Benefit bonus incentives can include promising individuals an additional half-day off if the organizationwide response rate is in excess of 80 percent or entering names of individuals who return surveys for a prize drawing.

Executive Responsibility

The chief executive officer or administrator of a health care organization has a distinct role in the survey process. The CEO takes the lead in communicating the survey and its directives to the entire organization.

One form this communication can take is the sending of an executive memorandum to all staff detailing the survey process and its objectives and encouraging all individuals to respond. Such an effort can be supported by CEO-led dialogue at staff meetings. In fact, many health care CEOs in the United States utilize such monthly "Friday forum" meetings to communicate directly to employees. In this type of open setting, employees can relay to the CEO what they have heard about the project, as well as any questions they might have. The CEO then has the opportunity to respond forthrightly and directly.

Any communication generated by the CEO, whether written or oral, should contain information clearly understandable by all individuals. First, the CEO must show complete support for the survey, reinforcing the notion that the survey is a good idea. If, after doing research, the CEO has any reservations about the survey, he or she should scrap the project. Without complete support from the CEO, a survey cannot be successful. Along these lines, the CEO makes an *action pledge* to try to meet the survey objectives and act on the results, including significant suggestions or recommendations that the respondents put forward.

The CEO also promises to provide the survey results directly to all respondents. The manner in which survey results are provided is secondary (whether by the survey team or by the CEO himself or herself, for example); the promise to provide them is primary. The action pledge should include the previously discussed time line for the survey process. The CEO reinforces his or her commitment to completing the survey by committing to, and staying within, the outlined time frame.

In addition to reinforcing the intended survey objectives and making an action plan, the CEO must assure employees of the confidentiality of the survey process. (Confidentiality must be a central theme in all communication relative to the survey.) He or she can communicate the promise of confidentiality initially in employee forums and in the hospital newsletter. The promise is reiterated in the cover letter placed with each survey instrument. This cover letter should contain the following components:

- A clear, concise statement of the survey's objectives
- An assurance of process confidentiality from collection and analysis through the action planning presentation
- An action pledge, indicating that appropriate action will be taken based on the survey's results
- An expression of appreciation to all organization members for participating in the survey process
- A statement informing employees of appropriate recourse they can take if they perceive any impropriety or major problem with the survey (the mode of recourse directs these types of problems directly to the CEO, who, in essence, has the main responsibility for the survey process)

The cover letter becomes a focal point in the survey process. It is an important practical information vehicle and emphasizes the importance of CEO commitment to the survey process.

Finally, there are other aspects of CEO communication. In the cover letter and in other correspondence and communication forums, the CEO can mention how the survey process will promote awareness of the organization's mission and quality improvement efforts. This subject may be particularly timely given that most organizations are presently involved in strengthening mission and values identification, as well as enhancing their continuous quality improvement (CQI) programs. Additionally, the CEO can alert employees that he or she has final approval of the actual survey. The fact that the CEO always maintains ultimate responsibility and authority for the survey gives the process a central focus and gravity. Furthermore, the CEO can communicate that he or she will monitor and examine all survey results. In fact, many CEOs state that they will participate in the survey themselves. This can help establish and/or strengthen a communication bridge between the CEO and all organization members. For example, when the CEO presents the results of the survey, if appropriate, he or she can reveal his or her own personal responses and explain how he or she "saw" the questions.

The role of the CEO is extremely important in the survey communication process. It sets the course of action, helps decrease negative sentiment, and presents a clear picture of the survey and its intentions. When the CEO takes the lead, all organization members feel that the survey is on the level and, therefore, a nonthreatening, progressive tool for organizational improvement.

Management Responsibilities

The commitment and participation of middle managers and supervisors are critical to the conduct of a successful attitude survey because this group has the most contact with employees. Therefore, these individuals are uniquely qualified to promote the survey and engage employee interest in the project. Figure 2-2 outlines the essential aspects of management participation in the survey process (planning, execution, and action planning). It is vital during the planning stage for all managers and supervisors to understand the intent of the survey. They help select the form and provide point-specific feedback relative to the construction and distribution of the survey. Because they have the most exposure to the employees, the middle line managers, along with their department supervisors, most directly communicate the intention and overall objectives of the survey. They also provide insight for the survey team into potential employee reaction and other dynamics that may affect the survey.

The survey conduct team can engage management participation by bringing managers in on every phase of the project. As with the line managers, a representative group of middle managers and supervisors attend short but pointed meetings on the survey and have the opportunity to review the survey instrument. They may be aware, for example, what particular word might

Figure 2-2. Management Participation in the Survey Process

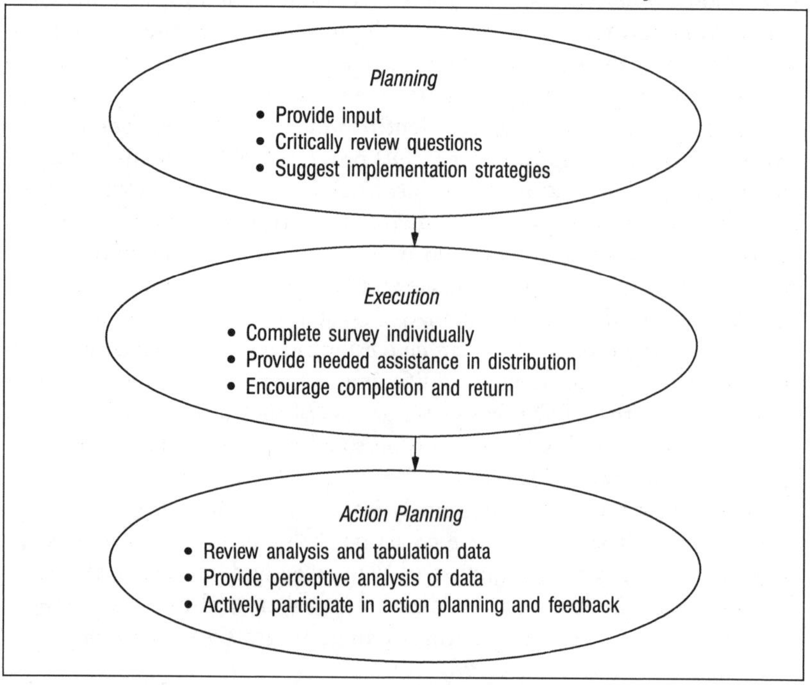

trigger a negative reaction, or a particular issue that might presently be affecting employee morale. By getting the support and participation of the management team, the survey conduct team heightens the participation level and positive employee and manager perception of the survey and increases the overall chances for success on the project.

It is important to note that the absolute, 100 percent full support of *all* managers is an impossible, if well-intentioned, objective. Some managers may strongly object to, or make arguments against, the survey for an assortment of reasons. However, it is important for the main survey conduct team to make every effort to engage overall support from the secondary management and supervisory team throughout the entire process. The following subsections discuss more specifically line managers' responsibilities, management forums, and key manager guidelines for survey success.

Responsibilities of Line Managers

The line managers' primary responsibilities are the promotion of the survey within their work groups and the gathering of feedback and support from the department members. To accomplish these tasks, the line manager utilizes six basic strategies:

1. *Open discussion in regular department meetings:* These meetings include participation of the survey conduct team and present basic survey concepts and desired objectives.
2. *Informal communication within the department:* For example, if an employee brings a positive and potentially valuable suggestion to the department head, the supervisor should not only make public note of the comment, but also encourage the employee to mention the idea in the survey.
3. *Employee focus groups:* Focus groups have been used successfully by many health care organizations. The most effective are those conducted by the manager in conjunction with the survey conduct team. For example, informal meetings no longer than 15 or 20 minutes are held in which employees are given the opportunity to review sample items or questions from the survey or to provide their own suggestions for items or questions to be included.
4. *Distribution of the surveys:* Managers should be involved in some form of survey distribution, as well as encouraging individuals to return the surveys once they have been completed.
5. *Participation in the survey:* The managers themselves fill out surveys. They should do so in a very visible manner. For example, managers can conduct an event (a luncheon, for example) at which managers fill the survey out in front of their employees.

6. *Continuous support of the survey:* The managers provide continuous visible support for the survey. They are the linchpin between executive management and employees.

The Management Forum

Many organizations utilize a management forum to focus specifically on the survey process for managers and supervisors. Again, a good communication vehicle is a management lunch (or ideally, two management lunches) that highlight the survey project. At one meeting, the initial survey agenda, general reactions, and immediate suggestions for improving survey effectiveness and efficiency should be discussed. At this meeting, the survey conduct team should take the lead, along with the CEO, in explaining the survey and underscoring its importance to everyone in the organization.

The second meeting is convened after the survey is completed. This final meeting is part of the action planning phase (discussed in more detail in chapter 5). At this second meeting, the managers review all survey results, comment openly about their perception of the results, and provide input to the subsequent action plan being developed.

Key Management Guidelines for Survey Success

As previously stated, management responsibility is key to the success of a survey. Any questions or apprehensions about the survey must be handled successfully in the planning process, and, through daily interaction with employees, the manager is responsible for maintaining the forward progression of the survey process. Following are some guidelines *all* line managers and supervisors can utilize:

- *The manager should understand that communication is key to the entire survey process.* He or she should communicate as openly as possible in order to involve everyone in the survey process. A manager should communicate any employee concerns directly to his or her superior and the survey conduct team. He or she should act as a listener, not only by gathering comments and suggestions, but also by gauging the attitude of the employee populace through simply picking up on any shifts in behavior or work patterns. Figure 2-3 summarizes the core communication roles of managers relative to employees and to the organization.
- *The manager should, throughout the entire survey process, fulfill the 10 basic roles of an "action agent:"*
  — Communicator
  — Distributor
  — Facilitator
  — Participator

—Monitor
—Consultant
—Reviewer
—Semiexpert on organizational issues
—Resource on prevailing employee sentiment
—Contributor to organization's progress

The manager explains the purpose of the survey and makes the initial foray into employee discussions relative to the survey's purpose and objectives. Subsequently, the manager must explain any particular aspects of the survey that might affect employee life, as well as clarify any mechanical concerns such as distribution and collection procedures.

- *The manager should be a living embodiment of the organization's commitment to use data generated by the survey.* Managers pledge their support to the survey process and reiterate to employees that any feedback and suggestions provided will be acted on, if appropriate, by both the organization and the manager.

Figure 2-3. Core Communication Roles of Managers

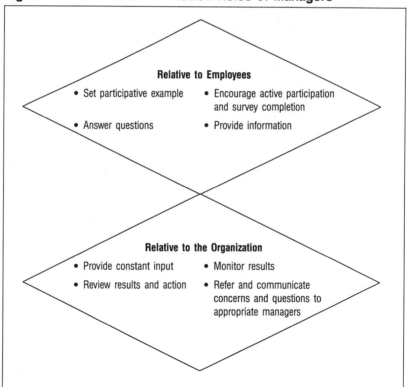

- *The manager should assure all employees that the survey is a "clean" process.* They should not take any action that might be seen as threatening or diminishing to the confidentiality of the survey. Managers should help maintain confidentiality of the process by proactively assuring all employees that the survey is aboveboard.
- *The manager should ask the right questions.* Asking the *right* questions of employees helps solicit their ideas and suggestions for the survey. Managers also ask questions of the survey team or senior managers to clarify their own personal viewpoints or perceptions of the survey and its objectives. Like the survey instrument, a manager can only be effective by asking the right questions at the right time.
- *Managers should stay involved in the survey process from start to finish.* Their involvement should include all of the roles displayed in figure 2-3 as well as three basic responsibilities:
  — The managers should encourage all individuals in the department and work group to fill out their surveys thoughtfully and to communicate openly with the survey conduct team and other individuals instrumental in constructing the final action plan.
  — The managers should express their commitment to the survey process through both words and action. Most important, they should express the "big-picture" relevance of the survey process and how it is vital to validating organizational direction and achievement.
  — The managers should impress upon all employees the responsibility that they all hold in the survey process and the importance of the instrument and the process itself.

By fulfilling their responsibilities to the survey process, the line managers and supervisors help accomplish survey objectives. Their involvement and interaction with staff generates a strong response rate as well as honest and varied responses. Furthermore, management participation helps fine-tune the instrument itself, increasing its effectiveness and efficiency. Finally, managers can ensure that the survey accurately reflects valid, prevailing viewpoints and perspectives.

Survey Instrument Construction

Defining planning objectives and communication responsibilities is only part of the survey process. The survey instrument itself is critical; content and/or mode of construction can trigger positive or negative reactions to it. Therefore, it is vital to ensure that the survey instrument meets various requirements for effectiveness and suitability relative to each particular organization.

The appendices at the end of this book suggest a survey system that has been used successfully by numerous health care organizations. The author strongly suggests that health care organizations utilize this system as a basis for constructing their own survey instruments in order to achieve a high response rate and collect meaningful data.

Essential Characteristics

A survey must contain certain characteristics if it is to be successful. These characteristics are:

- Consistency
- Clarity
- Inclusiveness
- Customer/patient focus
- Measurement of progress and the effects of change
- Commitment
- Resources supporting employees
- Continuity
- Comprehensiveness

Consistency

A successful survey instrument is consistent in terms of language, tone, and intent and must be the same for all levels of the organization, if possible. Variations in survey instruments can trigger misunderstandings or create suspicion, for example, when one individual sees that his or her survey is different from someone else's. The employee might make the erroneous assumption that he or she is somehow being targeted by management. Furthermore, it is vital for survey instruments to be consistent so that tabulation and analysis will also be consistent and meaningful.

Clarity

A survey must be clear. This means that the language on the survey must be understandable by all individuals using it. Additionally, all communication relative to the survey must be clear and concise. As previously discussed, individuals must know why the survey is being conducted and have a clear idea of its intentions, as well as its basic time parameters and other mechanical considerations. All of the issues engendered in the survey must be clearly defined and understood, not only by the survey team, but also by the respondents among employee and management groups.

Inclusiveness

The survey must be inclusive; that is, it must take into account the health care community at large. Nothing in the survey should lead to intentional destruction of group morale, organizational initiative, or unity among work groups. Words such as *we* and *our* must be used repeatedly in the survey, so that a sense of togetherness is reinforced. There should be no sense of finger pointing. A survey objective should be to help the organization become a more vibrant, positive entity within its community. This objective can be accomplished by addressing items that relate to the provision of services and the way in which those services are received throughout the community.

Customer/Patient Focus

The intent of the survey is to strengthen the organization in meeting the needs of the customer/patient, the most important person in the health care organization. Therefore, it is vital that some survey questions consider the customer/patient and his or her perception of the organization. For example, questions should ascertain whether survey respondents have the resources and support necessary to optimally serve the customer/patient. Such questions help respondents focus on the needs of the customer/patient, as well as show them that the organization is serious about improving customer/patient relations.

Measurement of Progress and the Effects of Change

The survey should measure progress and the effects of change. Its manner of construction helps employees focus on progress—both individual and organizational. A progressive well-motivated organization is a solid contributor to its community. Employees busy with their daily responsibilities often overlook this larger, important perspective.

By definition progress involves change, and every health care organization has had to deal with change at one point or another. The effect of change can be considered in terms of the past, the present, and the future. For example, the survey should inquire about any profound organizational changes that have taken place in the recent past. There should also be reference in the survey to changes currently taking place (particularly regarding new programs being implemented). Additionally, the survey should be a forum for discussing future change. This discussion would include determining whether employees have a good idea of what the organization's future plans are and their opinions in regards to them. The survey helps measure how change has affected various members of the organization and determine whether the change has had a positive or negative impact. Negative reaction to change hurts morale and can cripple progress. Positive reaction to change, on the other hand, reflects organizational growth.

Commitment

A characteristic of a well-constructed survey is measurement of employee commitment and perception of organization commitment to providing high-quality health care. Employees are aware of the commitment needed to maintain a strong health care organization. Though perhaps not formally (as in peer evaluation assessments), employees evaluate the commitment of their peers and coworkers on a daily basis. Most employees have distinct opinions about whether individual employees and the organization as a whole are committed to providing high-quality health care.

Survey questions can be posed in a nonthreatening manner to assist employees in expressing their opinions on commitment levels in the organization. A successful survey determines these levels because commitment is a major characteristic of an organization's attitudes and overall values.

Resources Supporting Employees

Because premier health care organizations seek to provide the best resources and support to all organization members, a survey should ask questions about resources (both emotional and practical) that support employees. Every individual should be given the opportunity to say whether he or she has all the resources needed to get the job done. Many organizations often overlook the fact that the employee actually performing a specific job is the hands-on expert in that particular job.

Consider the needs of an X-ray technician, for example. The technician knows specifically what type of equipment and resources are needed to perform his or her job on a daily basis. The technician also knows what support he or she needs from the supervisor. If the employee is unfairly hindered by a lack of resources or feels that there is better equipment or machinery, he or she should have the opportunity to present these thoughts clearly and openly. In the context of a manager–employee relationship, however, these types of conversations can be uncomfortable or inappropriate. Consequently, the survey becomes an excellent opportunity for the X-ray technician to address specific job role needs and assess the desire for future development.

Continuity

Continuity, the logical progression from objectives to actions, is important within a health care organization. All employees must be able to see a certain amount of synergy between organizational goals and actions. By utilizing the proper questions, a survey can help determine whether individuals perceive their organization as moving forward in a credible manner. All actions in a health care organization must lead to the common goal of providing high-quality health care.

Comprehensiveness

Finally, the survey must be comprehensive, taking into account all aspects of employee life. Specifically, the following five areas should be covered in a survey instrument (see also appendix A):

1. *The organization:* The entire organization should be assessed relative to the characteristics previously described in this subsection.
2. *The organization's management:* Management should be assessed in terms of direction provided, support given, and other aspects pertinent to a health care organization.
3. *The job:* Job specifics should be analyzed and assessed by the employee, and issues should be addressed relative to job conduct, growth, and professional development.
4. *The work environment/general issues:* Any current "hot" topic or organizationwide concern should be included in the survey. Employees should have the opportunity not only to comment on issues, but also to provide suggestions on how to deal with them.
5. *Management supplement:* In order to get a realistic view of the *entire* organization, the organization must make a specific effort to get managers and supervisors involved in the survey process. Therefore, a management supplement should be provided, which addresses issues relative to management concerns and supervisory responsibilities.

As just discussed, a survey must contain certain general characteristics in order for it to be successful. In the next subsection, constructing the specific elements of a survey instrument to incorporate these important characteristics will be addressed.

Survey Construction and Preparation

The survey provided in appendix A is divided into five sections: the organization, the organization's management, the job, the work environment/general issues, and a management supplement. This particular survey has been utilized with success in numerous health care organizations. It is important to understand *why* as well as *how* it works.

General Considerations

Any good survey instrument must have a sound format. The layout must be clear and understandable by all individuals. When a survey is constructed in five sections (as in appendix A), with a maximum of 10 statements in each, employee responses and opinions are garnered in a clean, crisp fashion. The clarity and directness of this construction help limit some employee concerns previously discussed, the fear of reprisal and a sense of suspicion, among others. The survey's physical appearance and a place for employee identification also bear on the project's success. The following subsections discuss these issues.

Section Construction
The 10 statements in each section are followed by a comments and suggestions section. The reason for this is that individuals will sometimes forget to

write down comments if there are more than 10 statements per section. Fewer than 10 statements per section gives the issues discussed in that segment an impression of insignificance. At the end of each set of statements, a section for general comments and suggestions is provided to encourage employees to address additional concerns and provide suggestions relative to the section. (See appendix A.)

A user-friendly format does not create undue pressure on the employee or become a job in and of itself. For example, in the late 1970s, the author worked with an organization that utilized a survey instrument containing over 150 questions. The survey took approximately 30 to 50 minutes to complete. Many of the questions were redundant or meaningless to the respondent.

The survey the author promotes in this book contains 50 questions clearly organized into five distinct sections and takes between 5 and 15 minutes to complete. The employees feel, therefore, that the organization values their opinion, but not at the expense of wasting their time or needlessly burdening them.

A user-friendly format broken down section by section helps employees focus on one specific area at a time (such as the organization or their particular job). By doing so, they are able to focus on key practical issues.

Physical Appearance

The survey instrument itself should be graphically appealing but not too extravagant. If the survey's appearance is not appealing, it may appear cheap, junky, or slipshod. Any negative impression suggests to the employee that the survey is not important. As a result, poor response rates may result.

On the other hand, if the survey looks too extravagant, employees may react apprehensively, and in some cases, open hostility may be generated. For example, if an organization is financially restricted due to budgetary or other concerns, the expenditure of several thousand dollars to print surveys in several different colors might appear to be a waste of resources. Each organization should utilize a style of survey presentation appropriate to its particular situation. However, most organizations can use an in-house desktop publishing program to make the survey look graphically appealing.

The survey needs a cover with the organization's name, logo, and the title "Organizational Survey System" or something similar on it. The internal printing should be clearly presented and free of typographical errors.

A letter from the CEO *must* be the first page of the survey. This letter reinforces the two important aspects of the survey—its importance and the promise of confidentiality. Additionally, in the letter, the CEO should pledge to provide survey feedback to all employees. This promise, as previously discussed in the text, must be supplemented by the commitment of managers and the survey conduct team to provide feedback in a timely manner.

Identification

A section should be provided for employee self-identification—shift, department, title, name, and contact information. This information makes the survey data more specific. However, a self-identification section should not be included in the survey unless the following proviso is also inserted: "Fill out any, all, or none of the below." The proviso reinforces the confidential nature of the survey but allows employees the opportunity to receive specific feedback and/or reinforce areas of the work experience that they have discussed in the survey through appropriate, voluntary identification that links their comments to a particular organizational component.

Appropriate Language

The language utilized in a survey is extremely important and therefore must be appropriately geared for survey success. As previously stated, the survey must be clear, direct, and easily comprehensible. As a general guideline, therefore, the comprehension language level should be set to a high school sophomore's level. Using this language level ensures that *all* survey respondents have a clear understanding of each item's intent.

The language in this book's model survey utilizes certain language dynamics. Whether or not an organization uses the model survey, it should be aware of these dynamics which, if used, will elicit strong survey response. First, statements, not open-ended questions, should be used. The responses to questions can be ambiguous, not lending themselves well to a straightforward result calculation. The statements should be somewhat general in context and yet focused on a specific organizational dynamic (see appendix A, the sample survey instrument). No statements should be misleading; that is, they should allow the employee to make a specific determination without leading him or her to a specific answer. Furthermore, if the questions are direct in nature, respondents are not forced to analyze the question's intent.

There are two language features survey statements must *not* use— absolute language and psychobabble. Absolute language includes words such as *never, always,* and *100 percent of the time.* Instead, the statements used in the survey should include terms such as *for the most part, in general,* and *usually.* These general phrases encourage the well-meaning employee to consider what usually happens in the organization rather than the rare instances when something out of the norm happened. For example, if a question such as, "In all cases, my suggestions are listened to," is used, even a well-intentioned, well-motivated employee may think of the one time that his or her supervisor did not "have time" to listen. Unfortunately, the 99 percent of the time that the supervisor did sit down and listen to suggestions is negated by the absolute nature of that particular question. A statement such as, "For the most part, my boss listens to my suggestions," is a more effective type of statement to utilize.

Survey language must avoid the use of "psychobabble," that is, psychological terms or groups of terms whose meanings are not easily understood. Often, when psychobabble is employed, respondents neither understand the question nor what it is "getting at." For example, if a statement reads, "Our work group shares information in a holistic manner," the average employee does not understand or misunderstands the question, or worse yet, dismisses the entire process as being an exercise in psychodynamics. The employee's opinion would be that the organization is "just trying to analyze us" or that management "does not live in the real world," because they are using terms on the survey that most employees do not employ regularly.

Instead, language that most individuals use daily should be utilized. The previous statement can be reconstructed as, "In most cases, our work group communicates openly and freely." This is a more direct, nonthreatening way of getting at the same issue.

Instructions and Scoring

The survey should contain instructions on how to fill it out, as well as a brief introduction at the beginning of each section, a deadline for completing the survey, instructions on returning the survey, and a source to contact if the individual has any questions. Among the instructions should be a brief note on how to complete the comments and suggestions sections at the bottom of each page. Also, all the basic instructions should be reiterated orally to the employees at survey distribution and collection.

The scoring system of the survey instrument itself is a matter of great importance. Respondents must understand the sliding scoring scale. Some survey planners like to use a seven- or ten-part scale. This is not advocated by the author, who proposes a five-part scale. The ten- and seven-part scales tend to reduce themselves to a five-part scale anyway, because individuals basically have one of five reactions to a survey statement. These reactions are:

- *Strongly agree:* Certain individuals will strongly agree with the content in a survey statement.
- *Agree:* On other questions, individuals will have basic agreement with the survey statement, described in terms such as, "for the most part, I agree with this statement."
- *Neutral:* Individuals who mark neutral to a survey statement have either no opinion, not enough information to take a definitive stand, or simply feel neutral on the issue.
- *Disagree:* This response indicates individuals have a basic level of disagreement with the statement. Disagreement registered at this level means that, "for the most part, I disagree with this statement."
- *Strongly disagree:* Individuals who select this response obviously have a strong reaction to the survey statement. The issue addressed is negatively affecting the respondent's work life and therefore the organization. Strong disagreement is a solid indicator of a potential problem within an organization.

As the analysis guides in appendix B indicate, the five-part scoring system works effectively in determining health care workers' and managers' attitudes. As long as a clear explanation is provided within the survey itself, most individuals find it an effective instrument in registering their opinions and attitudes.

The choices given to the respondents should be displayed as abbreviations (for example, SA or SD) rather than as numerical designations (such as 1) or alphabetical designations (such as *a*) that can lead to unnecessary confusion. It is burdensome and demotivating for employees already pressed for time to try constantly to remember what the scoring scale means. It can also cause inaccuracy in terms of survey data because employees can make mistakes in transcribing their answers. Also, the accuracy of survey data can been diminished when more than one scale is used. In these cases, the response rate is diminished because employees find filling out the survey to be "more trouble than it's worth."

Conclusion

This chapter focused on the planning and communication stages of conducting a successful survey. The actions discussed included the organization of planning objectives using survey planning meetings and time lines; the assignment of communication responsibilities at both the executive and management levels; and the construction of a sound survey instrument both in general character and practical specifics. By utilizing these suggestions and adapting particulars for individual institutions, an organization can construct a survey instrument that will not only encourage a high rate of return but, more important, provide meaningful, practical information.

Chapter 3

Survey Distribution, Collection, and Tabulation

Introduction

Once the organization completes survey planning, it is ready to distribute the survey to potential respondents. This chapter describes the distribution process, including specific distribution strategies and techniques for maximizing respondent participation and data generation. The importance of the collection process is also discussed, as are preliminary aspects of data analysis, including the tabulation of quantitative and qualitative responses.

Survey Distribution Strategies

The survey distribution process includes the printing of survey instruments and the administration of the surveys to potential respondents. (See chapter 6 for further discussion on printing the survey.) The distribution process usually takes between two and four weeks or a period of time adequate to afford all members of the organization the opportunity to participate in the survey process without feeling undue pressure.

There are two basic approaches to survey distribution: group and individual. In utilizing *group distribution processes,* organizations have employees complete the survey in group settings, thereby enabling quick collection and tabulation. Organizations wishing to further emphasize confidentiality and individuality utilize *individual distribution processes.*

When an organization considers which type of survey distribution process to employ, it gauges its interpersonal climate. For example, when there is a significant amount of employee suspicion or apprehension about the survey, the organization may decide to employ the individual distribution process. When, however, most employees work interdependently and are accustomed to group interaction, utilization of a group distribution process may be preferable. See figure 3-1 for a brief illustration of the pros and cons of group versus

Figure 3-1. Group versus Individual Distribution and Collection

Group Distribution	**Individual Distribution**
Pros	*Pros*
• Controlled environment	• Privacy and confidentiality maximized
• Guaranteed returns	• Specific comments enhanced
• Time management	• Independent thought encouraged
Cons	*Cons*
• Potential suspicion	• Lower return rate
• "Like" returns	• Possible manipulation
• Limited introspection	• Limited direction and return "encouragement"

individual distribution. The following subsections discuss the two distribution processes in more detail.

Group Distribution Processes

Through its community-type format, the group distribution process affords individuals the opportunity to participate in the survey process at a convenient time and, in many cases, in a comfortable setting. In any group process, clear instructions on how to complete the survey must be given by a member of the survey conduct team. Oftentimes to ensure confidentiality, the survey conduct team leaves the room once the employees have received the survey instrument and the instructions.

As stated previously in this book, the organization's goal in conducting a survey should be to achieve a high response rate *and* a high level of data quality. The following subsections discuss three settings for group distribution — at special meetings, at random meetings, and at regularly scheduled meetings.

Distribution at Special Meetings

The setting for the group distribution of surveys most often utilized by health care organizations is the special meeting. Organizations usually hold a series of meetings (often arranged as luncheons) devoted solely to the presentation and administration of employee surveys. For example, the process may begin with a luncheon for executive-level managers and their direct reports. At this first meeting, the survey conduct team describes survey goals and then distributes the survey instruments, which are to be completed by the end of the meeting. The managers thus have an opportunity not only to complete the survey themselves, but also to more fully comprehend the survey dynamics. With this understanding they will be better able to address survey-related questions from employees. When surveys are completed and collected at the end of a special meeting, a very high response rate is likely.

Immediately following the managers' meeting, a series of employees' meetings is conducted over the course of a week or two, depending on the size of the organization. At these meetings, the survey's intent is discussed, basic instructions on how to complete the survey are given, and then the instrument is distributed. A specific time period of approximately one hour is designated for employees to participate in the meeting activities (such as eating lunch) and completing the survey. Again, many organizations prefer this style of distribution because it almost guarantees a 90 percent or better response rate. Every employee except those who do not attend the meeting at least turns in a survey form, although some employees may choose to turn in incomplete or blank forms.

One might question, however, how accurate the results of a survey can be when it is distributed in a lunch meeting setting. Some employees might feel as though they are being monitored, and so their responses might not be as forthright as they would have been in another setting. Furthermore, employees may alter their responses to reflect those of others in their work group or those who happen to be sitting at the same table. Those conducting the survey need to keep in mind that the quality of response may be diminished owing to the dynamics of this particular group process even when the overall response rate is high.

However, there are positives to the employee luncheon distribution system. First, by treating the employees to a special lunch at the outset of the survey distribution process, the organization demonstrates its goodwill. Second, the word-of-mouth advertising generated by the first meeting is usually favorable. Most individuals in the organization (the 80 percent who are strong and steady players) generate positive comments about the survey. Third, as individuals see colleagues attending luncheon meetings, they feel more encouraged to contribute their opinions. Finally, when employees understand that all members of the organization *are* participating in the survey process, they recognize that *everyone* does have a vote in directing the organization's goals. Thus, they feel compelled to participate themselves.

Distribution at Random Meetings

Another group setting utilized by health care organizations is survey distribution at random meetings. In this format, the employee is afforded the opportunity to attend one of a number of specially scheduled meetings wherein the survey is discussed and presented by members of the survey conduct team and executive management. After the survey process is explained, the survey is completed by the employees. Approximately 20 to 30 half-hour meetings are presented throughout a given period (usually a week). All employees are notified about and given the opportunity to attend any meeting they wish. After attending a meeting and completing the survey, employees are asked to initial a sign-out sheet to ensure that no one fills out more than one survey. Many organizations prefer to distribute employee surveys at random meetings because the setting allows employees complete confidentiality in deciding when and where to complete the survey. However, when using this particular technique, an organization must provide opportunities for all employees to participate — night-shift, day-shift, off-site and on-site employees — in order to get a truly representative sample of the entire organization.

There are some drawbacks to this approach, however. Some employees may not feel motivated to attend any meeting, or some may have every intention of attending and then fail to do so owing to the demands of their jobs. Other individuals may feel uncomfortable because they fear that their responses will not be kept confidential or that they will be monitored in some way. Such concerns result in employee participation lower than it might have been if the organization had distributed the surveys individually.

Another consideration is that employees usually attend the meetings in self-selected groups. For example, opinions gathered from the night-shift workers in a respiratory therapy unit at an acute care hospital may be very different from those of other units or shifts. Or, at the same facility, various groups of nurses who attend different meetings may give the survey conduct team a terrific comparison/contrast of prevailing attitudes among the nursing staff as a whole. The way the employees attend the meetings and with whom they attend provide data in and of themselves.

An organization needs to be aware, however, that although certain employee groups may decide that it is a good idea to attend the survey meetings, others may discount the process as meaningless. Therefore, if the survey conduct team utilizes this process, it is imperative that managers and supervisors reinforce the efforts of the survey conduct team in "getting out the vote." Every effort should be made to encourage employees to attend and participate in one of the sessions. When all factors are considered, random employee meetings overall are an effective technique of garnering employee participation.

Distribution at Regularly Scheduled Meetings/Events

Group distribution can be incorporated into regularly scheduled employee–management activities. A monthly staff meeting in which employees review the survey for immediate completion or subsequent submission is the most typical and opportune example of this approach.

Some organizations, however, have used novel approaches to this idea. For example, one health care organization with whom the author worked utilized an annual baseball outing to obtain employee participation. Prior to boarding the buses provided by hospital management to take the employees to the ball park, individuals were asked to fill out a survey and drop it into a collection box. This approach may not work in every organization. The employees may see it as an infringement on their free time or, worse, as overt manipulation. However, in the author's experience, this strategy has worked very well, achieving a 91 percent response rate and a sampling of some very valid, diverse opinions and attitudes.

Organizations use various employee meetings or events to generate survey response. For example, at a regularly scheduled union meeting, attitude surveys can be distributed and then collected by the union representatives. These representatives then hand the completed surveys over to the survey conduct team. The author does not advocate this approach, however, because it is an unwieldy process to manage.

An organization must consider the following requirements when it utilizes a regularly scheduled meeting or event for group distribution of an employee survey:

- The process must be direct and manageable and require no more than a half hour for survey instructions, distribution, and completion. Otherwise, surveys may be misplaced or individuals may lose focus during the conduct of the regular meeting business.
- In order to ensure the validity of the survey process, at least one member of the conduct team must attend every meeting so that all questions can be answered and concerns resolved.
- All surveys must be collected before individuals leave the forum in which the surveys were distributed. Except in extreme cases (such as individuals being called away for medical emergencies), the survey should be completed and collected in the same room.
- Executive presence should be minimal when the employees are filling out the survey, and employee presence should be minimal when managers are filling out the survey. This allows individuals on the management team to fill out the management supplement freely and without distraction and employees to complete the survey without feeling as though management is monitoring their responses or using the survey in a manipulative or adversarial manner.
- The group process should encourage individuals and groups to attend the meetings randomly so that the survey process will not seem manipulative. Respondents should feel free to participate or not participate, as they wish.

Individual Distribution Processes

All factors considered, group distribution processes can be used effectively in gaining employee participation in the survey. However, most health care organizations prefer to use an individual survey distribution process for three reasons.

First, many health care employees' time is limited. They are already pressed to efficiently perform their job and personal responsibilities. Therefore, the group process can sometimes appear—and again perception is a very important reality in any health care human resources endeavor—to be burdensome.

Second, an individual process gives the employees more opportunity to consider their responses from their own perspective as opposed to a group perspective. In an individual approach, the individuals are not thinking about what their colleagues might be saying about the statements on the survey but are forming their own opinions.

Third, two important factors in achieving a successful survey—confidentiality and comfort—are often enhanced by the individual approach. The individual approach allows respondents to complete the survey in a place where they are physically comfortable, such as their homes or offices. These areas also provide individuals privacy. Additionally, in this type of setting, individuals can take their time to complete the survey; thus, their responses may be more considered and their comments more comprehensive. The following subsections discuss individual distribution processes in more detail— methods for monitoring individual participation and methods for distributing surveys to employees and members of the medical staff.

Methods for Monitoring Individual Participation

One of an organization's major concerns in utilizing individual distribution is that of control. Group distribution is a controlled process. The survey conduct team controls the number of survey instruments distributed and when and where employees and managers complete the surveys. Conversely, during an individual process distribution, it is difficult for survey team coordinators to ascertain how many surveys have been distributed and who has completed surveys. Therefore, organizations may utilize various control strategies. Implementation of these strategies have advantages as well as potential risks.

Coding
The most common strategy to control individual distribution is *coding,* that is, utilizing a code or marking to determine who is completing the surveys. Many organizations use a numerical code such as the employee's paycheck number or a specific number relative to their department and job position. For example, if the human resources department were considered the third group within an organization on an organizational chart and the compensation manager were the third-ranking member of the department, that individual's code would be 3-3. The advantage of such coding is that when surveys are returned, the organization has a good idea of who completed them. The disadvantage is that if employees recognize that a code has been attached to their survey, they will be more circumspect and perhaps less honest in their responses.

Some organizations utilize color coding. This strategy includes using color schemes to designate specific departments: pink for medical staff, purple for nursing, orange for operations, red for administration, and so forth. Individuals, however, can readily spot a code. Therefore, the employees may feel that their confidentiality has been compromised (even though this type of code is less specific than a numerical code).

Sign-In Sheets

Many organizations use other means of coding to determine whether individuals have completed the survey. A traditional approach is to have employees initial a sign-in sheet when they return their surveys. Employees can also sign in when they pick up their surveys. In this case, the survey conduct team can compare the sheets. Although who completed a survey is determined, names are not attached to particular surveys.

An obvious problem with this system is that individuals can sign in without actually returning a survey. The opposite problem also exists; that is, individuals may return the survey but forget to sign in. Finally, signing in may make some individuals feel that their confidentiality is being compromised. However, the sign-in system compromises the confidentiality of the survey process less than coding systems.

Tabs

Another method of monitoring survey distribution and completion is to attach a detachable *tab* to each survey, on the last page of the booklet, for example. After employees have completed the survey, they indicate their names and the date on the detachable tabs. They tear out the tabs and return the surveys at work or mail them back (depending on which collection strategy is used). The individual tab indicating survey completion is then mailed to or dropped off at a specific location. As with other monitoring strategies, the opportunity for inaccurate monitoring exists. Individuals can fill out the tab but not complete the survey or vice versa.

Other Methods

Some organizations utilize extra incentives for employees. For example, a small rural hospital used the tab method to monitor distribution. The tabs, returned separately from the surveys, were placed into a box situated in the hospital lobby. On the final date of survey collection, the CEO conducted a raffle drawing during which the top three winners received significant monetary prizes. This strategy was particularly effective at this hospital because most employees were genuinely interested in the survey and its results. There was very little manipulation of the survey return. This strategy, however, may not work at every hospital, particularly ones in which there is a significant amount of employee apprehension about the survey.

Another hospital also promised monetary prizes to individuals. These prices were given for the best suggestions under the "Comments and Suggestions" portion of the survey. At the end of the two-week collection period, the top 10 responses were presented to all the employees. The employees voted on which of the 10 were the best. In addition to the monetary reward, the winners received the reward of knowing their ideas were being considered for implementation.

Again, this strategy might not work at all hospitals, but this strategy, like the others presented, are at least worth an institution's consideration. It is incumbent on each organization to decide which, if any, of these methods for monitoring individual distribution processes is appropriate for the organization.

Methods for Distributing Surveys to Employees

Now that various methods for monitoring individual participation have been discussed, the different methods for individual distribution itself are explored. Methods of individual distribution utilized by health care organizations include the following:

- By mail
- Through polling
- In person
- With paychecks
- At random distribution points
- By executives
- By managers
- In phases
- Through employee committees

By Mail

One individual distribution strategy uses a mail system to distribute and collect the surveys. Most mail systems utilize a designated set of envelopes that give no appearance of coding or other potential threats to confidentiality. For example, many organizations mail the surveys to employees and enclose self-addressed stamped envelopes (SASEs) for survey return that show a post office box as the return address. The employee receives the survey and the SASE either at home or at his or her office. The employee then fills out the survey and mails the results to the post office box in the prestamped envelope.

This approach ensures confidentiality and underscores each employee's sense of his or her importance to the organization. When employees are sent surveys by mail, they tend to fill them out in a comfortable environment and to take their time and consider each question carefully. Employees tend to return the surveys in a timely fashion (within the allotted two weeks, for example) and usually give strong opinions and good insights. The response rate for these types of surveys is usually quite high. In fact, when the author recently conducted a survey using an individual mail system, he achieved an extraordinary 96 percent response rate. There was no magic potion that created this response rate — it was simply a matter of astutely matching (with the help of the hospital executives) the distribution strategy to the organization.

One shortcoming of the process is that the old excuse "it got lost in the mail" may be used, sometimes truthfully. Furthermore, some employees will not return surveys by mail if they are uncertain about who is receiving them. Obviously, it is incumbent upon the survey conduct team to assure everyone in the organization that the surveys will be returned to the survey team and not someone else in the organization. Finally, because Americans frequently receive mail surveys, employees may put the surveys aside to complete later on but never do so. As a result, the health care attitude survey may not be completed by many well-intentioned potential respondents.

Through Polling

Another individual distribution strategy is polling. Although uncommon, polling involves the execution of the survey in a one-on-one setting either over the telephone or in person. This strategy is often used by urban hospitals to conduct customer surveys.

However, when organizations use polling to conduct employee attitude surveys, the surveys can lose effectiveness. For example, when the survey is being conducted by someone whom the respondent feels is in a position of power over them, the respondent may not be as forthright as he or she would have been if he or she had completed the survey independently in a pen-and-paper format. Furthermore, there is potential for bias because of the interpretation and subjectivity of both the survey conductor (or pollster) and the respondent. The comments and suggestions elicited often can be generated more constructively and comprehensively in a pen-and-paper format because polling can degenerate into a conversation that provides less specific results.

Still, there are positive aspects to polling as an option for survey distribution. For example, respondents may understand more strongly the importance the organization has placed on the survey because the organization has discussed critical issues with each and every employee personally. Also, the respondent may provide more comprehensive comments in a conversational setting. Furthermore, important issues not addressed in a questionnaire may be uncovered by a skillful survey conductor.

Polling obviously takes a great deal of time and considerable expense when individuals are employed specifically to conduct the poll. However, this strategy is often effectively utilized as a follow-up process subsequent to the conduct of a traditional written survey.

In Person

Among the more traditional survey distribution strategies is survey conduct team distribution wherein every organization member is personally delivered a survey by a member of the survey conduct team. For example, for a 1,000-member organization, each member of the 10-member survey conduct team could distribute the survey to 100 employees. Personal distribution, when well organized, can be accomplished smoothly over the course of a day. When organizations use this strategy, it is common to see a large response rate within the first several days following distribution. The reason is simple—the personal distribution by the survey conduct team is a perfect complement to the comfort and confidentiality requirements for high survey response rate.

The in-person approach, however, has two minor problems. First, some individuals may be absent the day the survey conduct team presents and distributes the survey. Special effort should be made to get the survey to any individuals not in the workplace on the distribution date. Second, some individuals may be engaged in work activity and find the survey distribution an unwanted intrusion. Therefore, the survey conduct team should act thoughtfully when they deliver the surveys. Team members should keep a list of who has received the survey so that they can identify employees who have not yet received a survey.

A variation of this strategy is for human resources personnel to distribute the survey (survey conduct team members often work in human resources). In this case, the human resources department maintains the primary responsibility for distributing the survey to all organization members. This is accomplished by human resources personnel distributing the survey at a designated time on a particular day or asking employees to stop by the human resources office to pick up a survey. The latter is not endorsed by the author, as it creates an opportunity for many individuals to conveniently forget to pick up the survey and thus not participate in the survey process.

Another in-person strategy is for consultants from outside the organization to distribute the survey. This is the preferred method for unionized organizations and those that have experienced a significant amount of change. When a consultant distributes the survey, employee confidentiality and comfort are usually enhanced. However, if employees are apprehensive about the consultant as an individual or resent the intrusion of a third party into their organization, this distribution process may not be as successful as others.

With Paychecks

Paycheck distribution is a common individual survey distribution method. In organizations where paychecks are distributed every two weeks, the employee receives the survey in one paycheck and then in the next paycheck receives a gentle reminder about returning the survey. Paycheck distribution is particularly effective in large organizations and in institutions where there is a mood of cooperation about the survey. Paycheck distribution is not advised, however, in organizations where compensation is perceived as a problem or where benefits programs have been greatly restricted or reduced.

Random Distribution

Health care organizations also use random distribution. Random individual distribution involves placing large stacks of surveys at strategic locations within the hospital. The five most common areas include:

- The facility's main entrance or reception area
- The employees' entrance or the entrance immediately adjacent to the employees' parking lot
- The human resources department or an area outside the human resources office
- The employees' cafeteria or outside its entrance
- The conference rooms or auditoriums where employee groups meet regularly

Random distribution provides employees easy access to the survey forms, but it does not ensure maximum distribution. This distribution method does, however, provide maximum employee comfort and confidentiality.

By Executives

Another form of survey distribution used primarily in small hospitals is that of executive distribution. (In large health care organizations, this process might be somewhat difficult to manage because of the sheer numbers of employees compared to the number of executives.) In this process, senior executives distribute the survey to employees, usually on one predetermined day. The advantages of executive distribution are that the executives become involved in the process, thereby providing it with visibility and underscoring its importance.

Furthermore, when distributing surveys, the executives can take the time to communicate with the employees, answer questions, and resolve any problems concerning the survey process. There is one main drawback to this process: ironically, some employees may be intimidated by the very fact that the executives are distributing the survey.

By Managers

In large organizations, manager-to-employee distribution can be utilized to accomplish the same objectives as executive distribution. In this process, department-level managers and supervisors distribute survey forms to their employees. Distribution can be done in the context of a regularly scheduled departmental meeting or a specially convened meeting in which the survey is discussed, its deadline for completion set, and the processes for returning the survey for collection and tabulation explained. In these sessions, questions can be answered relative to the survey and concerns can be resolved by managers. A manager-to-employee distribution process works effectively in a large organization because of the close contact many supervisors have with their employees as well as the ratio of managers to employees. As with executive distribution, opportunity is presented for managers and employees to discuss issues and to become actively involved in the survey process, thus increasing the level as well as the quality of response.

In Phases

In staggered distribution, the health care organization distributes the surveys in a phase-by-phase process. This means, for example, that some departments receive the surveys on one day and other departments receive the surveys on another. The survey conduct team is able to gather information clusters on particular departments. Survey distribution in phases helps to manage the survey process in large organizations (2,000 or more employees), where a great number of people will be completing the survey.

The disadvantage of staggered survey distribution is that it can create management problems within the survey process. For example, there have to be two or three collection processes rather than just one. Additionally, individuals may feel that their department is being slighted because their surveys were distributed at a later date. Again, staggered distribution is only recommended in organizations that are large because of the potential for employee distrust and negative perception of the survey process.

Through Employee Committees

A form of survey distribution is the utilization of an employee committee. That is, a designated group of employees (usually volunteers) distributes the surveys to colleagues at a prescribed time. This idea has particular appeal in organizations in which employees are actively involved and truly interested in the results of a survey. When this strategy is used, the volunteers simply pick up surveys from the survey conduct team and distribute them to a designated work group. Employees may distribute surveys to their own work group or to others. The latter method allows employees to learn a little about different departments in the organization, thereby increasing interdepartmental communication. Furthermore, this strategy encourages confidentiality, especially when individuals distribute surveys to departments with whom they have little contact.

Methods for Distributing Surveys to the Medical Staff

Depending on its organizational structure, the health care institution may wish to give not only employees but also physicians and other affiliated professionals the opportunity to participate in the survey process. Such organizational partners often provide useful input and suggestions. A survey conduct team can use any of the employee distribution methods suggested in the previous sections to get the partners' input. However, the most effective strategy to utilize is having a designated member of the survey conduct team distribute surveys specifically to physicians and other affiliates. This individual manages the entire distribution and collection process and, in many cases, keeps the surveys separate from those of the general employee population. Because physicians and other affiliated professionals play unique roles in the organization (and therefore have a unique perspective of the organization), their data should be kept distinct and separate. However, these data are critical and usually provide useful insights.

Survey Collection Strategies

It is essential for those conducting the survey to understand that the collection process starts with the distribution process. When surveys are distributed, all instructions for collection should also be publicized. Key concepts in the collection process are *convenience* and *confidentiality;* that is, all employees should have the opportunity to return the surveys in a manner that is convenient to their work schedules and ensures utmost confidentiality. This section discusses both group and individual collection strategies.

Systems for Collecting Surveys Distributed to Groups

If any type of group distribution process is utilized (such as an employee lunch), then the surveys should be collected at the end of that session. This is accomplished by requiring all respondents to place the completed forms in a designated box or envelope. It is the responsibility of a survey conduct team member to be in charge of this collection box or envelope.

Systems for Collecting Surveys Distributed to Individuals

The collection process is a seemingly mechanical one, but it is extremely important to the success of the survey project. As previously stated, confidentiality and convenience must be the keystones of the process, enhanced by logical action and open and ongoing communication. Each health care organization should choose the collection strategy that will most effectively achieve these objectives for itself. (See also chapter 6.) Regardless of which collection process is utilized, six basic keys should be kept in mind:

1. Designate a specific time and place for collection, either noting several times and places where the employees may return the survey or reiterating the method for mailing in returns or other strategies. Clear communication is critical to this process.
2. Allow a week grace period after the designated deadline during which individuals may return the survey. This would be accomplished by using a letter and/or other reminder mechanisms to allow individuals "one last chance" to return the survey. This grace period often increases the

response rate as well as response quality because some individuals simply are too busy to complete the survey while others simply need to see their colleagues do something first before they attempt it themselves.

3. Involve a union representative in the collection process. It is most important in union situations that a labor representative (such as a shop steward or other individual) is an ally in the collection process. Even if the individual feels as though the survey is a perfect opportunity for employees to register their "gripes" with management, it is better to keep this communication aboveboard than have it occur in a subversive manner.

4. Ensure that there is closure in the collection process. Utilize the survey conduct team, particularly the employee members, to remind individuals about the deadline. Once the surveys have been collected, the survey conduct team generates word-of-mouth notice that the survey has been completed and the results are currently being tabulated and analyzed. This ensures that all organization members know that the process has reached the end of one phase and is progressing toward a positive conclusion as promised.

5. Remind people of the cutoff dates and keep communication open throughout the collection process. This might include, for example, managers reminding members of their department about the survey or notice given in individual paychecks and other organizational communication relative to returning the surveys.

6. Ensure that some sort of postcollection mechanism is in place (that is, that any late returns can be submitted) and that there is a process following the conclusion of the actual survey to collect comments generated by the survey. Individuals may have ideas, comments, and suggestions they did not feel were appropriate to submit on the survey itself. The survey conduct team should encourage these individuals, as well as the management of the health care facility, to present additional comments and suggestions in either written or verbal form to a survey conduct team member, the human resources department, or an appropriate manager.

The collection process should include the generation of a letter by the CEO or the survey conduct team that serves as a friendly reminder about returning the survey. For example, if the survey is distributed on October 1 and the targeted collection date is October 15, the survey instrument specifies that the survey should be completed and returned by October 15. The CEO's reminder letter should be sent out on October 12. This letter reminds individuals to return the surveys by the 15th but also indicates that the collection boxes or other survey collection mechanisms will be in place until October 20, allowing for late returns.

Many survey collection techniques define the distribution techniques. For example, if a mailing strategy is used to distribute the survey, a mailing strategy would be used to collect the survey (return envelopes are provided in the survey). However, as with the distribution techniques, it is imperative that each organization utilize the collection system that makes the most sense for it in terms of liability and potential effectiveness. The following subsections discuss some of these techniques.

Direct Collection

Direct collection by the survey conduct team is often used. The survey conduct team acts as a neutral party specifically to collect the surveys from all respondents. Collection can be done on a designated date and completed within a day or two of regular work time. This approach is positive in that it is relatively effective and extends a personal touch to the collection process. On the other hand, *because* the surveys are collected personally by a member of the survey conduct team, some respondents, fearing a lack of confidentiality, may feel apprehensive about returning the survey.

Collection Boxes

Currently, most health care organizations favor using a collection box system because this process ensures convenience and a sense of confidentiality for employees. Collection boxes are usually placed at five strategic areas throughout the facility (the same places where surveys were distributed in an open distribution)—in the main lobby or reception area of the facility, at employees' entrances, by access doors to the employees' parking lot, near the employees' cafeteria, and outside the human resources department. The collection boxes should be sealed. Some organizations put locks on boxes, and others use cardboard boxes clearly sealed with strong masking tape. When the survey boxes are finally opened, it is done on the designated collection date in full view of employees and other people passing by. This process assures skeptical employees that the surveys have been collected in a fair, responsible manner.

It is equally important to note that even if an organization uses a mailing system, it maintains a collection box philosophy. Some hospitals have made the mistake of having individuals mail surveys back to the facility, notably the human resources department. The problem with this strategy can be that individuals fear that the human resources department is collating the surveys in an effort to identify respondents or groups of respondents. Accordingly, a good solution is to utilize a post office box in a town immediately adjacent to the hospital or health care facility. The address of the post office box should appear clearly on the SASE in which the survey is to be returned. The address also should be highlighted in the CEO's letter in the survey instrument. This ensures confidentiality and lends further anonymity to the survey process.

A variation on this collection box strategy is the utilization of preexisting suggestion boxes. Suggestion boxes are logical places either to return surveys or to place specific survey collection boxes next to. In either case, as long as the boxes are clearly marked (for example, with "Employee Survey Collection Box"), confusion about where to return the surveys should not ensue.

Unfortunately, given the state of labor relations in some health care organizations, it is important to emphasize collection box security. In some organizations, it is effective to utilize a wooden box with a padlock to preclude any tampering with the survey process. Unfortunately, some individuals may try to reproduce surveys and stuff the box or, as is more often the case, remove surveys from collection boxes. It is a good idea to have security personnel keep an eye on the survey collection boxes to prevent such tampering. Furthermore, individuals apprehensive about theft or tampering can be reassured that their survey will be in good hands until review by responsible parties.

Collection by the Human Resources Department

The human resources department in health care organizations can be utilized as the main collection point. This collection strategy is most effective in small facilities or in institutions where the human resources department is viewed by employees as a positive, progressive presence. In these cases, the human resources department maintains the collection boxes or utilizes a large file cabinet to collect the completed surveys. Once the surveys have been returned to a designated department representative, he or she locks the surveys in a box, or file drawer. Each organization must examine its current political climate before utilizing this technique. Its advantages are the expansion of the role of the human resources department in a very important organizational process and the utilization of the human resources department as a catalyst in achieving a high response rate.

Public Collection

When utilizing a public collection strategy, the survey conduct team organizes a group of employee volunteers to assist in survey collection. For two or three successive days, these volunteers set up tables and collection boxes in the front of the lobby and at the entrance to the employees' cafeteria. During designated hours (for example, at lunchtime or at shift changes), the collection teams will be in place. The employee volunteers simply collect the surveys from their colleagues and place them in a box during these designated periods. Also, a member of the survey conduct team is on hand at each site at all times.

The advantages of public collection are clear. By involving the employees in this critical stage of the process, good word-of-mouth communication about returning the surveys is generated throughout the organization.

Furthermore, a certain amount of positive peer pressure can be exerted to encourage individuals to return the survey. Also, because employees tend to trust each other, confidentiality, comfort, and convenience are enhanced.

This particular process has a few potential negatives. Managers may feel uncomfortable in returning the survey to an employee or certain employees may fear that a fellow employee will read the survey prior to placing it in the box.

To alleviate the first problem, the institution should organize a collection process exclusively for managers along the same lines as that for employees. For example, management surveys can be collected at a management meeting or at a specified time in an executive conference room. To alleviate the second problem, employees mistrusting each other, the institution can allow employees themselves to place their completed surveys directly into the boxes as opposed to handing them to fellow employees.

Survey Tabulation Strategies

Once the surveys have been distributed and collected, the tabulation process begins. All of the completed forms are looked at from a quantitative and qualitative perspective. This section discusses the tabulation process, with specific emphasis on the system presented in appendix B of this book.

Tabulation begins as soon as the collection process is completed. The sooner results are tabulated, the sooner analysis can commence. Some organizations use *random sampling tabulation;* that is, they take a representative sample of responses to determine data outcome. For example, if 500 surveys were returned, only 200 surveys would be randomly selected and tabulated for use as a representative sample of the entire organization.

Other organizations advocate *universal tabulation;* that is, all data in each and every survey are included in the tabulation. Every survey is analyzed and every response considered in determining the overall survey results.

The universal process reflects prevailing employee opinion accurately and precisely. However, most industrial psychologists believe that in any organization of significant size (200 or more employees), a 50 percent random sample provides an accurate reflection of the entire organization. In either case, health care institutions should tabulate surveys numerically and collect all significant comments and suggestions respondents provide on the survey instrument.

Tabulation guides are provided in appendix B for each question within the survey. However, it is also important during actual tabulation for individuals to try to analyze specific trends or patterns. For example, are there any patterns in the responses to the survey? Many individuals may mark "neutral" to a particular question. Tabulators make a note of this type of trend by keeping a notebook handy during the tabulation process. (This notebook will provide further data for analysis.) Other types of patterns may appear. For example, it is not uncommon to see in succession several groups of employees responding the same way to a particular question. This can mean that several employees completed the surveys together or it can mean that many employees feel the same way about a particular topic. Again, this finding should be noted.

Quantitative Tabulation

The tabulation process begins with a *quantitative tabulation*. If an organization uses the process suggested in this book, the collected surveys are organized into five piles. The stacks are organized by survey sections—organization, management, job, work environment/general issues, and management supplement. Numbers are calculated to achieve percentage responses for each question (see figure 3-2).

A significant number in the survey process—in fact the first computation to be made—is the overall response rate percentage. According to most industrial psychologists, a good response rate is 60 percent or better. Sixty percent or better is indeed a very good response rate in a health care institution, considering the amount of activity and emergency situations handled in a given day by the average health care professional.

After the overall response rate has been determined, data are tabulated according to shift, department, professional type (nurse, technician, and so on), full- or part-time status, and any other pertinent subcategory. Subcategories can include and of the following:

- Department
- Job
- Shift
- Length of service
- Full- or part-time status
- Union participation

Figure 3-2. Percentage Conversion Method

Section II, Question 5, Responses:

Strongly Agree	Agree	Neutral	Disagree	Strongly Disagree
43	153	21	70	56

Percentage Conversion (Each response rate divided by total response rate):

Strongly Agree	Agree	Neutral	Disagree	Strongly Disagree
13%	45%	6%	20%	16%

- Physical location within the organization (if multifacility organization)
- On-site or off-site location
- Any suborganization, such as a division, clinic, or other designation
- Name

In some organizations, individuals may be hesitant to designate name, shift, department, and so on, as requested on the last sheet of the survey. *Whatever* information is provided, the individuals tabulating the surveys should feel free to make notes on the survey instruments. Handwritten notes allow quick and easy access to information.

Personal knowledge also should be part of tabulation. For example, any specific concerns of certain individuals known by the members of the survey conduct team should be addressed. Furthermore, individuals have different perspectives on issues. The tabulators should also be aware of the following factors:

- Employees' length of time in the organization
- Employees' organizational level
- Employees' job position
- Employees' length of time in current position
- Employees' promotional opportunities
- Employees' exempt/nonexempt job status
- Employees' sex
- Employees' age
- Employees' ethnic or cultural type
- Employees' domicile (within/outside of service community)
- Groups affected by change
- New departments
- Department's physical location in the building
- Major amount of change within the department
- An old "established" department

Any of these variables, if known to members of the survey conduct team, should be noted on the survey.

Qualitative Tabulation

The second part of tabulation is *qualitative*. Qualitative tabulation consists of looking at *all* comments and suggestions written by respondents. For every stack of at least 100 responses, any 5 or more similar comments or suggestions should be considered significant. The tabulators should accurately paraphrase significant comments and suggestions into their notebooks. When survey analysis takes place, these comments and suggestions should be considered.

Other significant information tabulators should enter into their note-books includes:

- Positive suggestions that might have immediate rewards
- Citations of particular individuals by name for positive actions
- Citations of particular individuals by name for alleged negative, illegal, and/or highly unethical actions
- Allegations of unethical or questionable actions against a manager or a group of employees (even if a strong "clue" but no name is provided)
- Reiterations of issues already addressed in the survey
- Citations of specific incidents that have been especially troubling to employees
- Citations of specific incidents of which the employees are particularly proud

Using their judgment, the CEO and other responsible executives will develop strategies in the action plan to address these issues. (See chapter 5.)

As in quantitative tabulation, the survey conduct team must stay cognizant of commonalities in the qualitative tabulation. For example, several surveys may contain the same comments. Employees may have gotten together in the interest of expressing a point to the survey conduct team. These individuals are probably very curious, to say the least, about what management will do with their "feedback." It is important that one note not only these comments, but how they were received. For example, one hospital used a collection box in which the collected surveys landed in a perfectly balanced stack. It was easy to distinguish the employees who got together when preparing responses because all their surveys arrived at the same time and contained largely the same suggestions. Although the author does not advocate the use of such collection boxes, it is important to collate information in such a way that it can be easily referenced, grouping similar comments and suggestions together (whether positive or negative) for further analysis.

When conducting qualitative analysis, the survey conduct team should read between the lines. Some individuals may make no comments or suggestions whatsoever. For example, in 10 recent health care attitude surveys conducted by the author, the average number of surveys returned with comments and suggestions was approximately 35 percent. Also, tabulators should note surveys that provide a multitude of comments and suggestions. Certain individuals may attach additional sheets or write their extensive comments on the back of the survey. Tabulators should note not only comments and suggestions, but the intensity with which they were offered.

Tabulators should also look for any unusual characteristics in the completed surveys. For example, when many individuals return surveys stapled shut, this is a sign that employees anticipate reprisals for giving honest feedback. For the same reason, some individuals may type their responses so that their handwriting cannot be identified.

It is important for the survey conduct team to pay attention to any such clues that the tabulation process can provide. The clues help produce more accurate and meaningful data and therefore provide more positive survey outcome.

Conclusion

Distribution, collection, and tabulation transform a survey from concept into reality. These processes must ensure the comfort, confidentiality, and convenience of the respondents and the accuracy of the data. This chapter addressed some ways to manage these processes for optimum survey results. As in every phase of the survey project, each health care institution's survey conduct team must utilize its business instincts and common sense to make these critical processes effective and efficient within the context of each organization's culture.

Critical Analysis

Introduction

After the survey data have been tabulated, critical data analysis and action planning can begin. Most members of the organization, in addition to feeling curious about the numbers and percentages generated by the survey, are very interested in the future plans the organization decides to establish on the basis of the survey results. Therefore, the survey team must conduct a thoughtful analysis to guide the executive management team in preparing an appropriate action plan. Critical analysis is discussed in this chapter; action planning in chapter 5.

The analysis phase of the survey project must be undertaken in a logical manner with a great deal of introspection. All survey conduct team members and others involved in the analysis (such as designated executives, consultants, and the human resources staff) must look into the *why* as well as the *what* behind the survey results. This chapter provides the insight and practical tools needed to analyze survey results thoroughly and thoughtfully with the goal, as previously noted, of providing positive change and progressive action for the institution. The areas of analysis discussed are quantitative analysis, qualitative analysis, and interpretative analysis.

Quantitative Analysis

Survey tabulation begins with numerical or *quantitative analysis*. Several factors must be considered when compiling a quantitative analysis. First, the numbers should be accurate and show no evidence of tampering. Second, the numbers should not be slanted to support any predetermined conclusions. Essentially, there must be *no* guesswork. Any conclusions must be based strictly on the data provided by the survey respondents. There should be a clear correlation between the numerical responses and any conclusions or recommendations made by the survey conduct team or senior management. Quantitative analysis is tabulated on both an overall and an item-by-item basis.

Overall Response Rates

The first survey finding to be analyzed is the *response rate* or the *return rate*. As stated in chapter 3, many industrial psychologists believe that a successful organizational survey is one that generates a response rate of 60 percent or better. A strong response rate can usually be attributed to good survey mechanics. The higher the response rate, the more the organization can claim that the results of the survey represent a majority opinion or the "employees' vote." Such majority of opinion, therefore, helps executives gain consensus support for future plans. As discussed throughout this text, the survey that the author advocates generates a response rate that is significantly higher than 60 percent. Many conditions, however, affect the survey response rate.

If an organization's survey response rate is higher than 65 percent, the following factors may have contributed:

- Organizationwide interest in the survey
- Recent changes within the organization
- Effective use of survey dynamics
- Strong management support
- Solid survey instrument design
- Positive employee interaction and word of mouth
- Presence of a strong development department or employee education department
- Strong employee and management desire to participate

On the other hand, a response rate of less than 65 percent may indicate a certain amount of negativity and low employee morale in the organization. Reasons why the response rate may be less than 65 percent include:

- Poor application of survey dynamics from the outset of the survey project
- Widespread suspicion that precluded individuals from answering in a forthright manner or participating at all
- Presence of a third party (such as a union) that did not encourage individuals to complete the survey (or, worse, discouraged them by using fear tactics)
- A certain large group of employees (such as a nurses) that did not participate at a significant rate
- Fear of reprisal
- Inadequate collection mechanisms perceived by the employees to diminish confidentiality (such as coding or collection box misplacement)

- Addressing of items in the survey considered by employees to be irrelevant or intrusive
- Utilization of too many feedback instruments in the organization (such as a previous survey within the past calendar year)
- Misunderstanding of the survey's purpose, format, language, or objectives
- General employee apathy toward all organizational activities (including low morale and a lack of positive motivation within work groups)
- Major changes within the organization (such as layoffs or reorganizations) that have left individuals feeling insecure
- Major activity within the organization that kept individuals too busy to complete and return the survey within a designated time frame
- Poor word-of-mouth communication generated by the employees relative to the survey
- Antipathy or mistrust relative to the relationship between upper management and the employee population throughout the organization

A response rate of less than 65 percent, however, should not be considered a damaging blow to the organization's morale. As we have seen, there are many reasons why the response rate to a survey project may be relatively low. However, these reasons require more numerical definition. For example, any response rate greater than 50 percent indicates a simple majority response from the organization—essentially, a successful survey return. Any response rate greater than 40 percent represents a plurality in the strictest numerical sense and again can be somewhat representative of the overall organizational population. However, any response rate of less than 40 percent is poor and probably indicates major problems within the organization. Using 40 percent as a threshold, the organization must identify the dynamics relative to a response rate that is either lower or higher than that critical number.

Item-by-Item Analysis

In conducting an item-by-item analysis, one compares specific items and determines why one statement triggered a stronger reaction than another. For example, if communication is a key issue within a health care organization, the survey items related to that issue might have been "strongly disagreed" with at a significant rate.

Even when the responses are negative on an item-by-item basis (that is, there was a certain amount of disagreement or strong disagreement to positively positioned statements), it is better for the organization to know and thereby respond to the prevalence of these feelings. Otherwise, negative sentiments continue to fester.

Appendix B demonstrates how to conduct a thorough, item-by-item analysis. It provides analysis guides for every item in the sample survey instrument provided in appendix A, along with specific instructions on using the guides.

Specific Response Rates

Whenever possible, response rates are broken down according to specific demographic groups (discussed in chapter 3). Given certain shift requirements, department compositions, and other factors, one generates and analyzes numbers on a group-by-group basis. For example, if a significant number of individuals from a given department responded, that response data could be analyzed on a group basis. Specifically, if 200 employees worked in the maintenance, plant engineering, and housekeeping departments of a community hospital (under the overall designation of environmental services), 100 or more identifiable responses would represent a majority within this work group. Individual responses are tabulated, after which common group trends and concerns are identified. This information helps the director of environmental services and his or her staff to construct a departmental action plan and specifically to understand the attitudes and critical issues relative to that specific work group.

Group-based data are also compared to each other and to data from the organization as a whole. For example, one particularly crucial interdepartmental comparison is that of shifts. Individuals who work on the night shift often handle diverse responsibilities and operate under conditions quite different from their day-shift peers. In many community health care organizations, the nursing supervisor on the night shift acts as a de facto administrator. This is due to the large amount of night-shift activity and the absence of traditional departmental supervisors, who usually work on an eight-to-five schedule. Individuals who work on the night shift may have very different opinions and concerns than those on the day shift. Therefore, as much as possible, a survey should try to identify respondents by shift and make comparisons where appropriate and useful.

Another area of comparison is between union and nonunion employees. It is very difficult, however, to separate these two groups of employees during a survey project. Often, labor laws and other contract dynamics do not allow individuals to identify themselves as union or nonunion employees on a survey, even on the identification page. However, many individuals utilize the survey's comment and suggestion segments to identify themselves as union or nonunion members to make a specific point. In conducting survey analysis, management should use such information thoughtfully and constructively.

Pockets of Response

Finally, in compiling a quantitative analysis, one must try to identify *pockets of response,* that is, identify any group of employees that responds in a similar fashion in a seeming effort to send management a message. For example, at a hospital where the author assisted in conducting a customer survey, many individuals from a specific part of the community answered in a similar fashion. They lived in a part of the city in which certain hospital services were to be eliminated. They felt the elimination of these health care services would be detrimental to their community. The individuals' pocket of response became clear with their strong disagreement to a specific set of statements on the survey. The survey conduct team analyzed these responses and then presented the results to executive management. These data encouraged the executive management team to reconsider its pending action, and the team ultimately changed their course of action relative to proposed services elimination.

Survey analyzers identify pockets of response by looking at the numbers of "like groups" of respondents, those from similar departments, demographic groups, shifts, and so on. As in all quantitative analysis, the numbers must be valid in order for the survey to be considered credible. In other words, one tabulates the numbers of categories or subgroups *only* when such groups are clearly identifiable.

All data should be prepared by utilizing the basic steps outlined in appendix B and listed in a clear, concise fashion. Figure 4-1 illustrates a basic scoreboard. This type of scoreboard can be used in the analysis of data and as a demonstration tool to share information with managers and employees during the postsurvey meetings. The clarity of these tables can assist executive management and the survey conduct team in comparing the survey data in order to make conclusions and recommendations.

Figure 4-1. Scoreboard Format for Survey Responses

Table A: Management Response—Section I/Organization

Issue	Strongly Agree	Agree	Neutral	Disagree	Strongly Disagree
1. Work atmosphere	25%	68%	4%	2%	1%
2. Preparedness	14%	57%	19%	10%	0%
3. Ethical action	31%	59%	9%	1%	0%
4. Growth plans	18%	61%	14%	7%	0%
5. Communication	7%	32%	31%	28%	2%
6. Employee input	3%	41%	33%	21%	2%
7. Employee selection	13%	69%	16%	2%	0%
8. Positive perception	33%	57%	10%	0%	0%
9. Responsiveness	15%	70%	12%	3%	0%
10. General position	12%	65%	13%	10%	0%

Qualitative Analysis

Not only are the surveys analyzed quantitatively, they are analyzed qualitatively. In *qualitative analysis,* those analyzing survey results focus on the employees' comments and suggestions. The qualitative analysis works in concert with the quantitative analysis to provide further insight into issues and trends of concern to employees.

In the tabulation process, all comments and suggestions are separated from the quantitative data. As previously suggested, any specific comments and suggestions appearing with a high rate of frequency are tabulated. In the planning process, the survey conduct team and executive management make a decision as to the definition of "frequency." Some health care organizations consider any five similar comments within a survey "batch" of 100 to be significant; other organizations consider similar comments and suggestions from 10 respondents out of 100 to be significant. Each health care organization establishes its own appropriate "frequency" baseline. The establishment of baselines is predicated on the following criteria:

- *The number of individuals within the organization:* If an organization has fewer than 500 employees, any comment that appears on 15 or more surveys out of 300, for example, is considered significant.
- *The nature of the comment:* If the comment applies to a group dynamic (such as general compensation or total quality improvement throughout the organization), the frequency should be set at 5 responses or more. In most organizations, critical issues usually have more than 5 responses within a batch of 100.
- *The nature of the comment itself:* If the comment is positive and supported by 10 or more responses in a group of 500, for example, the comment is noted as significant. Extremely negative or extremely positive comments are also highlighted, regardless of the number of similar responses.

This last comment touches on a very important characteristic of qualitative analysis. Certain comments and suggestions that appear on the survey are included in the qualitative analysis despite level of frequency or support from other respondents. Comments and suggestions falling into these categories are always highlighted and subsequently directed to senior management in a timely fashion:

- Comments alluding to unethical actions within the organization, such as illegal practices or questionable medical care
- Comments questioning certain business practices (in addition to those that are considered unethical), including ineffective methods or incidences of noncompliance

- Comments referring to a specific crisis situation the respondent feels the survey has not addressed, such as faulty equipment or other operational mechanisms
- Comments citing personality conflicts that are hampering performance and causing psychological distress for the respondent
- Comments citing any actions of a discriminatory or harassing nature
- Comments acknowledging a fellow employee's performance "above and beyond the call of duty"
- Viable, sensible suggestions for a specific action that will positively affect the organization
- Comments reinforcing ideas or strategies the organization uses
- Comments reflecting potentially negative major change within the organization, such as potential union issues, which should be discussed in the briefing session
- Suggestions for significant operational improvements heretofore not discussed or considered by management
- Comments from the community the health care organization serves that can have specific relevance to the organization's objectives

Primarily, the qualitative analysis is a process through which data that may be helpful in making an organization a more effective health care provider are collected and tabulated. The following characteristics of the comments and suggestions must be considered:

- Viability
- Validity
- Intention
- Relevance
- Objectivity

Viability

All comments and suggestions should be viable. Many health care professionals know exactly what they need to get their jobs done but often *want* more than the organization can provide. Therefore, those analyzing the survey should dismiss any suggestions that seem to be unrealistic or simply outside of the boundaries of practical application. For example, many individuals may suggest that the organization buy another hospital or renovate the entire building. These and/or other suggestions simply may not be financially viable for the organization. Often, the employee is aware that his or her suggestion is unrealistic and is simply venting his or her frustration.

Validity

The validity of all comments and suggestions should be analyzed by the survey conduct team. That is, in the judgment of the team, is the comment true or false? For example, some disgruntled employee wishing to throw a wrench into the survey process may make false accusations about discrimination, harassment, or other potentially explosive issues. Such information must always be considered seriously. However, the first question the survey conduct team and executive management group must ask themselves is, "Is this for real?" If the comment appears to be valid, it must be acted on immediately. An investigation is composed of two steps. First, the accusing individual (if identifiable) is questioned by executive management and asked, in a confidential way, to discuss his or her comments. Often, when an individual has not identified himself or herself, the comment is found to be false. The second step of an investigation involves the human resources department looking into any allegations or negative comments to determine their relative validity.

The validity of comments can also be related to inaccurate perceptions on the part of employees. Their perceptions *are* their reality and therefore should be addressed. For example, in a metropolitan hospital, many respondents may state on the survey that "because the hospital is losing money, it is impossible for me to do my job." Such comments alert senior management to further open communication with employees. In this case, a senior management executive, preferably the CEO, takes it upon himself or herself to present a financial overview of the hospital as part of the briefing. Whether the hospital is actually losing money, that is the perception of the concerned employees, and it must be addressed.

The greater the frequency of comments, whether valid or invalid, the more the issue should be addressed. Comments are reviewed by the survey conduct team and addressed by senior management in the postsurvey all-staff meetings and other actions subsequent to the survey.

Intention

The survey conduct team members must ask themselves why an individual might make a specific comment or suggestion; that is, what is the employee's intention? Among the motives for making suggestions are these:

- To get back at someone
- To make a point
- To deliver a message
- To misguide the survey conduct team
- To create a false impression
- To try to indicate to senior management anger over an issue

- To indicate overall dissatisfaction with the organization
- To "have fun" with the survey instrument
- To express honest interest in having comments heard and acted on

Only comments made for the last reason should be acted on. If the intention of the individual is truly to make a positive change within the organization or to correct a negative organizational action, the survey conduct team should note the comment as significant and prepare an action plan or route the comment to the appropriate person. Although the first eight motives should not be ignored, they are more properly addressed by the human resources department, not the survey conduct team. The human resources department should address those motives in concert with ongoing operational development and management development efforts.

Relevance

When reviewing comments and suggestions, the survey conduct team should be attuned to the statements' relevance. Individuals often make comments and suggestions on the survey that are irrelevant to the organization or its present status. Individuals may make suggestions on the survey that have nothing to do with the provision of health care. For example, one individual commented on a survey that many service organizations provide customer inducements such as two-for-one opportunities in purchasing goods. This comment is irrelevant; it is difficult to imagine a medical staff providing operations on a two-for-one basis. In another case, an individual noted that nurses were treated unfairly at her particular hospital because the school-teachers in a community 60 miles south of the hospital were paid considerably better than the hospital's nurses were. Obviously, this comment was not relative to the issues at hand: although teaching and nursing are similar in some ways, they are two different professions. The survey conduct team, composed of a cross section of individuals from the organization, will have the experience and knowledge to determine whether a comment is relevant.

Objectivity

In qualitative survey analysis, objective comments must be distinguished from subjective comments. Fundamentally, individuals respond subjectively. That is, they respond emotionally, especially to issues important to them. It is with these issues (for example, job training or lack of equipment) that individuals will usually be overly subjective, often writing extra comments and suggestions on the survey. On the other hand, individuals are usually more objective when discussing issues that do not hit home so closely. For example, the organization's future growth, though pertinent to many, does not have as much impact on the employees' daily lives as their relationships with the immediate supervisors.

When looking for subjectivity during a quality analysis, the tabulators must focus on three basic areas:

- *Tone:* positive or negative as represented by the language utilized
- *Content:* length and basic opinion
- *Focus:* specific issues and objectives that the individual is addressing

The consideration of these three factors in overall survey analysis cannot be underestimated. By following their instincts and using common sense, the survey conduct team can make positive use of all qualitative analysis data.

Interpretative Analysis

Once quantitative and qualitative analyses are complete — the data checked for viability, validity, intention, relevance, and objectivity — *interpretive analysis* begins. As the name suggests, interpretative analysis consists of making certain interpretations and conclusions relative to the survey data. This type of analysis is always risky. In order that the survey conduct team and the executive management group not read too much into the data, they should utilize the author's 10 basic guidelines when doing interpretative analysis. The guidelines call for them to check the data for:

1. Validation
2. Revelation
3. Innovation
4. Invention
5. Ratification
6. Indignation
7. Protestation
8. Supposition
9. Castigation
10. Rationalization

The first five are positive reactions; the next four negative. Rationalization provides the "why" for all.

Interpretative analysis takes advantage of the education and professional knowledge members of the survey conduct team and senior management group bring to an organization. This analysis helps these groups formulate the promised action plan. (See figure 4-2.)

Figure 4-2. Interpretative Analysis Elements

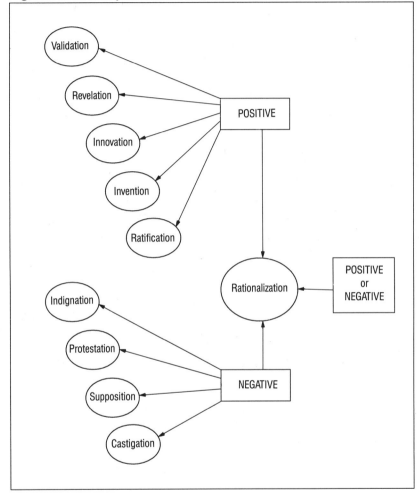

Validation

A *validation* is any opinion and/or insight offered by respondents that concurs with senior management's prevailing assessment of the organization. For example, in one organization many managers and employees may feel that intraorganizational communication could be improved. This perception is validated as reality if most survey questions relative to communication indicate that such a communications problem does indeed exist.

From the outset of the survey process, it should be made clear that the survey is a tool to validate what executive management, along with the survey conduct team, consider to be the organization's strengths and weaknesses. The survey conduct team and senior management (as previously stated), along with some middle managers, line managers, and supervisors through various CQI efforts determine the assumptions to be validated. This can be achieved by first making some specific statements or assumptions generally agreed to be on target. Figure 4-3 is an example of an organization's list of validations. Throughout the course of the interpretative analysis, the survey conduct team seeks significant data, comments, and suggestions supporting these validations.

Revelation

Revelations include any unanticipated data or comments arising out of the survey process. Revelations about negative *and* positive actions should be noted and acted on as necessary. For example, a certain comment may alert the organization to a heretofore unknown unethical action ongoing in a particular department.

. However, the survey conduct team must be careful not to fall into the trap of looking only for negative revelations. Revelations can also be positive in nature. For example, an employee may cite the work or effort of a fellow employee that contributes to the good of the hospital but was unknown to other individuals. Revelations, both positive and negative, are fundamental to the construction of a strong action plan.

Innovation

Any employee comment suggesting new, progressive action that would utilize existing organizational resources is an *innovation.* For example, an individual may offer the answer to a facility's parking shortage by suggesting the utilization of land or other space the hospital already owns. Another

Figure 4-3. Example of "Top 10" Management-Held Validations List

- Many employees have seen their job roles expand dramatically
- Our benefits package should be examined for possible "enhancement"
- The recent failed union attempt left some people very bitter
- Most people in the organization enjoy their jobs here
- The physicians "get along" with everyone else
- Most members of the organization are excited by the new construction project
- Most organization members think more parking is needed
- Our customer/patients are treated with the highest level of service in all regards
- New services are implemented smoothly and effectively
- In general, people here believe that we are "ready for the future"

innovation may be the utilization of a different financial mechanism to decrease billing delays.

Individuals with technical expertise often conceive innovations. The survey is an opportunity for them to make suggestions that might help increase not only their own work productivity, but also the organization's overall work quality. As noted often in the text, individuals should have been strongly encouraged to use the survey in this fashion. When innovations are suggested, it is then the responsibility of the survey conduct team to decide the viability of implementation.

Invention

Invention in interpretative analysis is closely related to innovation. An *invention* is a brand-new process or procedure that requires more resources and fiscal expenditures than an innovation. It also needs resources and materials not currently present in the organization. For example, the inventive answer to the problem discussed in the previous section may be purchasing additional land for parking. The inventive answer to the fiscal dilemma may be to implement a new computer system in the hospital.

Useful inventions must be reasonable and practical. Often, the survey conduct team does not have the expertise necessary to determine whether an invention is practical. Therefore, the survey team routes the ideas to the individuals in the organization with appropriate knowledge. In doing so, the survey conduct team does not inadvertently leave good ideas by the wayside.

Ratification

A *ratification* is a comment or suggestion made by an employee that indicates basic approval of organizational direction but does so more specifically than a validation. In section I of the sample survey in appendix A under Organization, several statements refer to the organization's movement and its future action plans. Here employees have the opportunity to express their opinions on these issues.

Ratifications may appear in other areas of the survey. For example, employees may ratify on a departmental or individual basis approval of leadership. Any ratifications indicated are included in the survey analysis report because they emphasize tangible positives in the organization. Unfortunately, there is a tendency among survey conduct teams to ignore ratifications and focus unduly on negative reactions.

Indignation

There are negative reactions, however, that the survey conduct team should record in an interpretative analysis. The first is *indignation*. Any comment registered on the survey addressing the loss of an employee's or an employee group's dignity should be recorded by the survey conduct team and addressed by executive management as quickly as possible. Employees may register indignation at their treatment (or that of others) by other employees, by a certain manager, by the entire organization, or by customer/patients.

Many employee comments that register indignation within the context of a survey fall into two categories. The first category is *meaningless indignation* wherein an individual is letting off steam about a situation that is actually not a problem for an overwhelming majority of employees. In this case, the indignation must be perceived as divisive venting.

The second category is *positive indignation*. Even though an individual is expressing indignation, he or she is also providing a solution (either explicit or implied) for resolving the dilemma. For example, because health care professionals deal with people in crisis situations and have close interpersonal contact with customer/patients, visitors, and peers, they are very sensitive to inappropriate interpersonal communication. For example, a well-meaning health care manager may use a term he or she does not realize is offensive to an ethnic minority. Accordingly, if indignation toward an individual's comments is registered on the survey, the problem can be easily remedied by the survey conduct team. In this case, appropriate action consists of educating the individual or the individual's manager with the help of a human resources specialist as to the appropriate language to use so as not to show disrespect (however inadvertently) to others.

The survey conduct team records expressions of indignation that appear on surveys. However, the team always considers the intention and credibility of the comments and uses common sense when addressing any negative issues.

Protestation

Protestation is another negative emotional reaction recorded by employees on the survey. Protestations are usually made by employees disgruntled by the organization overall. These employees use the data responses as well as the sections for comments and suggestions to protest against an individual or a particular organizational action. The survey conduct team should consider protestations with caution. Often, it is only a single person venting on a very specific issue or letting off steam in general.

For survey tabulators, a good rule of thumb in reviewing protestations is to be aware of their frequency. That is, if several individuals within a work group or any other significant number of individuals register the same protest, the survey conduct team must attach validity to the comment. To return to the parking dilemma, for example, perhaps administration has recently rerouted employee parking to ease congestion and traffic. If 1 or 2 individuals out of 500 complain about the rerouting, most seasoned health care managers and executives would agree that the administration has done a fine job in rerouting the parking, given the normal incendiary nature of this type of change. However, if 30 out of the 500 individuals register a complaint, the survey conduct team can assume that other individuals are dissatisfied as well. In an organization, 30 out of 500 individuals is a significant percentage. In this case, the protestation should be recorded and addressed by senior management as soon as possible.

Supposition

Supposition in interpretative analysis includes any rumors, innuendos, or conjectures supported by survey comments. Suppositions take the form of the following types of comments:

- "The hospital is losing money, therefore. . . ."
- "The hospital is going to lay off several people soon, therefore. . . ."
- "The administration does not care about our department, therefore. . . ."
- "Soon we are going to be bought out by hospital X, therefore. . . ."

As these examples illustrate, two negative dynamics occur in supposition. First, if a supposition is widely held (whether true or false) it may affect performance, as reinforced by the second aspect of supposition, the "and therefore" dilemma. Rumor almost always stimulates negative responses. For example, several surveys may record like responses such as, "The hospital is losing money, therefore we should be worried about our jobs." The rumor has resulted in employees fearing loss of their jobs, obviously lowering morale.

It is the survey conduct team's responsibility to record all suppositions. This is particularly important when any supposition is held by more than one employee. The team must first assess the validity of the supposition and, if it is merely a rumor, clear it up. For example, if a widely held supposition is that "the hospital is losing money," the senior executive conducting the post-survey debriefing meeting might distribute, if appropriate, copies of the hospital's recent financial statements that show that the hospital is not losing money but, in fact, is doing quite well financially. Suppositions can be exacerbated if not addressed during the survey process. The survey conduct team and the organization's senior management must ensure that in the survey debriefing process all rumors are nipped in the bud. If this is not done, the individuals may turn to their colleagues and say: "See, it must be true. We talked about it on the survey, and they didn't want to answer it. Therefore, management must be really scared because they would not even address the situation."

Castigation

Castigation can be interpreted from a survey response any time criticism is leveled directly by the survey respondent at the organization or at a particular segment of the organization (such as senior management). Castigations usually take the form of very direct, anonymous comments, and their direct, specifically-focused nature is what differentiates them from protestations. In fact, the stronger the castigation, the less likely that the survey respondent will be to sign his or her name or provide any other critical personal information.

The survey conduct team should record all castigations and then review them thoughtfully. The tone and focus of the castigations are clues as to their sources. In some cases, castigations might have validity. If an individual complains about another by name, the one being castigated should be informed with appropriate tact and confidentiality by the appropriate person. This should be done in a manner that does not compromise the confidentiality of the survey process and the rights of the survey respondent. However, it is also the right of the individual who is being castigated to have at least the knowledge that someone has a very strong negative opinion about his or her performance. The survey responses of individuals employing this type of strategy are usually negative in their entirety.

Rationalization

Finally, the survey conduct team records any rationalizations that appear on the survey. *Rationalizations* include any comments in which an individual explains why he or she feels so strongly about an issue or a person. In other words, rationalizations provide the answer to the question "why."

Rationalizations can be positive or negative. The survey conduct team should acknowledge any rationalizations as important (particularly when they are given by more than one person). Any subjective comment provided on the survey that is offered to explain a response further is a rationalization.

Conclusion

The analysis phase of the survey project—composed of three parts: quantitative, qualitative, and interpretive—is critical to the survey's success. As this chapter discussed, analysis must be conducted thoughtfully and clearly, utilizing the experience and knowledge of the survey conduct team members and any reviewing executive managers. The more comprehensive the analysis, the more sound the subsequent action. By utilizing the information in this chapter in concert with the analysis guides contained in appendix B, this objective can be fully realized.

Chapter 5

Action Planning

Introduction

After the survey results have been carefully analyzed (as discussed in the preceding chapter), the last phase of the survey process—action planning—is undertaken. The organization's assets and problems identified by the survey respondents suggest the direction for positive change on four levels— organizational, departmental, environmental, and individual. Indeed, for the survey process to be successful, its effects should be felt throughout the institution.

If the change process is to be meaningful and widely accepted, some actions must be undertaken immediately after the survey results have been analyzed. After the survey conduct team and the senior management group identify specific problems (for example, shortcomings in the employee benefits program), they communicate with the individuals or departments affected (in this example, the human resources department). They also communicate positive comments immediately to the appropriate person and investigate reports of unethical or unprofessional behavior without delay. Such direct actions show the respondents that their comments and suggestions have been and are being taken seriously by the survey conduct team and top-level management. In addition, preliminary survey results and plans for future meetings on the subject are communicated as appropriate to individual department managers and interested groups within the organization.

After organizational, departmental, environmental, and individual action planning is complete, the action plan is presented to the entire organization in an informational meeting or a series of meetings during which further input from all members of the organization is encouraged. These meetings, conducted by top-level managers and members of the survey conduct team, emphasize positive action planning rather than further venting of complaints.

After the action plan has been refined according to comments made in the informational meetings, the organization is ready to implement the plan over an appropriate period of time. Positive, long-term change predicated on the survey results will incorporate initiatives aimed at solving problems as well as programs designed to implement new ideas and support already-successful processes and individual contributions.

Planning for Immediate Action

As soon as the analysis phase of the survey project has been completed, some of the areas identified by survey results need to be translated into immediate action. Significant comments and suggestions that have specific application within the organization should be acted on before further longer-term action planning is initiated. The areas to be addressed immediately include communication of positive comments and simple suggestions, communication of negative comments, and utilization of employee–management review committees. In addition, soon after survey data have been analyzed, preliminary action plans are formulated by executive managers and members of the survey conduct team with direct input from the managers and work groups affected by the plans.

Communication of Positive Comments and Simple Suggestions

Immediately after the analysis phase, the survey conduct team and top-level management relay any specific information identified to the individuals or departments directly affected. For example, if a respondent cited the strong, positive contributions of a fellow health care worker, the cited individual should be informed of the compliment without delay. Or, if the survey identified a specific problem in a technical department or patient care unit that might be easily remedied by a suggested action, the problem and suggested solution should be relayed for immediate consideration directly to the individual in charge of the department or unit. As another example, perhaps several respondents indicated that the emergency department's admitting procedures could be made more efficient by slightly modifying the initial reception process. In this case, the suggestion would be conveyed immediately to the emergency department director because it has the potential to increase the efficiency of the department.

Next, the survey conduct team and senior management address problems identified by a significant number of respondents. For example, if 60 of 200 total respondents complained about a specific element of the facility's employee benefits package, the survey conduct team should immediately alert the human resources department that there may be a problem with the employee benefits package.

Informing the human resources department serves two purposes. First, the department receives feedback that may help remedy a problem or at least promote understanding of what a number of employees perceive as a problem. Second, giving and acting on immediate feedback adds to the survey process's credibility. That is, the human resources department is given an opportunity to remedy a problem (or at least to investigate a potential problem) and the executive management team and the survey conduct team note this when presenting the action plans. Employee respondents then see that their input *is* valued and is resulting in positive organizational change.

The survey conduct team members and executive managers must always keep in mind that the department managers and technical experts are the true authorities in determining whether suggested changes, innovations, and inventions have merit. Accordingly, the survey conduct team forwards specific recommendations directly to the individuals most able to accurately determine their viability.

Again, the primary benefit of routing specific suggestions to appropriate individuals for consideration is that organizational progress can be achieved quickly and positive change can be fostered. The secondary benefit is that the employees are assured that their suggestions were referred to individuals in a position to take immediate action. Furthermore, they can be encouraged in the postsurvey informational meetings to follow up on their suggestions with coworkers who are already aware of their ideas.

Communication of Negative Comments

Any potentially negative or destructive comments are also acted on immediately. Negative comments include specific allegations of unethical behavior or illegal activities as well as any actions that may cause immediate harm to the organization or to its customer/patients, employees, or medical staff. Again, the survey conduct team is not the best judge of the potential danger. Negative comments are directed to the individuals who have the most understanding of control in resolving the problem (for example, the chief executive officer [CEO], the department manager, or the director of human resources). The survey conduct team looks to its senior member to decide specifically to whom the negative comments should be routed. For example, if a suggestion of general sexual harassment within the workplace were raised, the human resources department and appropriate legal counsel should be brought into the matter. To give another example, if there were a report of racial prejudice against a specific manager, the CEO might need to be notified in addition to the human resources director, and appropriate legal counsel.

Taking immediate action to address problems suggested by negative comments is crucial to the survey's success. Respondents take a significant risk by registering complaints in the survey. The trust that they have placed in the instrument and the organization may be destroyed if their comments are not investigated and, if appropriate, acted on. In the all-staff informational meetings held after initial action planning, it is imperative that the CEO acknowledge negative comments and provide information about how they were investigated and resolved. This not only assures the individual respondents that their comments were taken seriously, but also assures *all* members of the organization that negative situations, once identified, will not be allowed to continue.

Because all negative comments are investigated, even those that ultimately prove false are quickly addressed. For example, an allegation of misconduct against an executive could be investigated and proved to be unwarranted. Then in the staff meetings, the CEO could reveal that an allegation of misconduct registered on the survey was investigated and found to be groundless. In this way, false accusations can be discouraged without suggesting that legitimate negative comments are unwelcome.

Employee–Management Review Committees

Another immediate action strategy is the utilization of *employee–management committees* (also called *survey review committees*) to review the data analyzed and compiled by the survey conduct team. The committee may be made up of individuals who have not so far participated actively in the survey process. Committees may play several important roles at this stage in the survey process because they act as:

- Focus groups that review and discuss the basic ideas arising from comments and suggestions expressed in the survey
- Reaction groups that look through survey data and responses and report on their immediate reactions
- Conduits for information sharing with the appropriate parties when action from either positive or negative comments must be acted on immediately
- Sources of supplementary data that enhance survey comments and outcomes
- Advisory boards that present survey data and outcomes to the organization

The committees can make specific suggestions as well as report to the survey conduct team what committee members have been hearing from other employees about the survey. Such information thus helps the survey conduct team understand the effectiveness of the survey project at the same time it supplies valuable information for fine-tuning the action plan and the format for the postsurvey all-staff meetings.

Communication of Preliminary Results and Future Meeting Dates

Finally, the survey conduct team makes a preliminary report of its findings to the executive management team, principally the CEO and his or her direct reports. This presentation includes information on the general trends and outcomes of the survey. It also includes a short (five-page) overview of the survey results. The overview includes the numerical data findings from all five sections of the survey instrument, augmented by summaries of the comments and significant suggestions made by respondents.

The preliminary report is also offered to representatives of any significant employee groups, such as unions. In a nonunion setting, the report may be given to specific employee committees. Then, in addition to disseminating information about the survey's outcomes, these groups generate some positive word-of-mouth and give the survey results valuable publicity.

As a last step in the immediate action phase, the survey conduct team generates a memo, signed by the CEO, that explains to all organization members when and how the postsurvey meetings will be conducted. In addition to the memo, information on the postsurvey meetings is released in employee newsletters and other in-house publications. Usually, postsurvey meetings are held about a month after the survey collection deadline. This allows the survey conduct team enough time to analyze the data completely and take whatever immediate action is called for in response to the survey.

Finally, at this stage, the survey conduct team can take additional immediate action on anything that makes sense to them. For example, some organizations have communicated the numerical results of the survey to the whole organization immediately after the data were compiled. This strategy may work well in small organizations, particularly when the results are largely positive. However, it may backfire in large organizations because staff may have less interest in attending the postsurvey meeting when they already have seen the basic survey results. Obviously, when the results of the survey are mostly negative, it would be foolish to distribute them without explanation before the postsurvey meeting.

Planning for Long-Term Change

After planning for immediate action in response to survey results, action planning for long-term change within the organization is undertaken. This action planning entails a detailed executive review of the survey results and a thorough impact analysis. The four main areas of action planning are:

- *Organizational action planning:* This covers planning for changes in the organization as a whole, including changes in its management and leadership systems.
- *Departmental action planning:* This covers planning for actions that affect individual departments, units, and other work groups within the organization.
- *Environmental action planning:* This covers planning for improvements in customer relations and the organization's responsiveness to the surrounding community's needs.
- *Individual employee action planning:* This covers planning for changes and problem solving to improve individual output and morale.

Organizational Action Planning

Organizational action planning begins with an analysis of the responses given in sections I and II of the survey instrument. (The whole survey is reproduced in appendix A and analysis guides for sections I through IV are provided in appendix B.) These sections explore the characteristics of the organization as a whole as well as the organization's management and ask respondents for ratings in several key areas.

The survey conduct team and executive management incorporate the following as part of their impact analysis and action planning:

- Any new plans developed for organizational improvement
- Any plans directly linked to comments and suggestions provided by the survey respondents
- Any measures to be taken to combat negative situations identified by the survey and strategies to enhance positive attributes emphasized in the survey

By communicating such information in postsurvey all-staff meetings, the management team lets employees know that their voices have been heard and, more important, that their advice will be heeded.

Formulation of Issue and Action Statements

Many organizations, as evident in the sample organizational plan reproduced in appendix D, utilize a specific format for formulating action plans that result from impact analyses. Key issues, such as organizational communication (issue 1 in the sample plan), and the possible actions to be taken in response to those issues will be described. It is important for the survey conduct team and executive management to utilize a format that first allows assessment of the survey results, then identification of specific issues, and finally creation of strategies to resolve problems and enhance positive actions.

Formulation of issue and action statements in organizational action planning include exploring:

- Management communication
- Morale and motivation
- Management strengths and abilities

Management Communication

One area of management to be examined is communication, that is, the direction and feedback provided to employees within the organization as a whole. The amount, content, clarity, and consistency of communication generated by the organization are considered in reviewing section I results. In addition to the specific points suggested in the analysis guides (see appendix B), the comments and suggestions in section I responses are also considered. Recommended actions related to communication are then formulated. (Again, refer to appendix D for an example.)

Morale and Motivation

Another organizational consideration involves overall employee morale and motivation. This issue appears in several areas of the survey, and it is an important touchstone in terms of putting together an action plan. The organization's human resources and education departments should be involved in the development of an action plan for this area.

Management Strengths and Abilities

An assessment of the survey respondents' overall perspective on the strengths and abilities of the organization's management are also considered in impact analysis and action planning. An objective of the executive management group and the survey conduct team is to examine the effectiveness of not only the organization as a whole but also of the managers who run it. Survey results provide many clues that suggest management effectiveness. For example, an indicator of divisiveness may be the respondents' use of the pronouns *us* and *they* in discussing employee and management groups. Although it is important to avoid reading too much into the us–they perspective, all are encouraged to utilize a collective *we* throughout the postsurvey all-staff meetings and subsequent management communications.

Review of New Ideas and Suggestions

Any new ideas and suggestions relevant to the organization as a whole are reviewed, and their validity is assessed, along with their potential for adoption. When management decides that an idea will be implemented, they credit the idea's originator and publicize the adoption of the idea in the postsurvey meetings. When a new idea is not considered valid and/or viable, this decision is also discussed at the meetings. Indeed, feedback is given to everyone who made suggestions, and all employees are encouraged to suggest other ideas in the near future.

Departmental Action Planning

One of the most critical aspects of action planning for long-term change is departmental action planning, that is, incorporation of survey results into action plans relative to specific departments and work groups. When data are examined on a group-by-group basis, in conjunction with department managers, executive managers, and members of the survey conduct team, specific action plans are constructed that make an organization more productive. Furthermore, the survey becomes an invaluable tool to the department manager in maximizing performance and optimizing the department's contribution to the organization.

Throughout the course of the survey, many individuals identify their particular work group, either explicitly on the information page or implicitly by the nature of their comments. Accordingly, fairly accurate assumptions can be made about the attitudes of specific groups. Action plans can then be formulated with specific work groups or departments in mind.

Role of the Department Manager

The central element of group and departmental analysis and action planning is the participation of the manager or supervisor. The department- or unit-level manager or supervisor participates from the outset of the analysis process when the survey conduct team has collected substantial information about a department or work group. The manager is able to offer unique insights about why specific comments and suggestions may have been made. He or she is also the organization's technical expert in action planning for the department or work group.

Many survey questions relate directly to the management of a specific department as perceived by the survey respondents. Indeed, in the survey instrument illustrated in this book, an entire section is dedicated to this subject (section II). Although many respondents may not feel comfortable citing the work of their immediate managers, many do when they feel as though the impact of the managers' work is directly affecting the achievements of the work group.

Because department managers and supervisors should understand how they are perceived by their employees, managers from all organizational levels should be involved in the process of action planning for improvements in management systems. To accomplish this objective, the survey conduct team works with the executive who manages several department managers or supervisors. The executive manager is made aware of the specific ratings that his or her reports received on the survey. A group-by-group analysis is then conducted on each of the executive manager's departments or work groups. The executive reviews any specific action plans suggested by the respondents and makes additional suggestions about possible departmental action plans. Then, depending on the style of the organization, the executive manager discusses, either in conjunction with the survey conduct team or in a one-on-one setting, these plans with the specific department managers. In these meetings, the department managers are given the opportunity to respond to the survey data, including assessing employee credibility and possible bias and the viability of the employees' suggestions and comments.

Formulation of Issue and Action Statements

Figure 5-1 shows an example of an issue and action statement that pertains to two specific hospital departments. The subject is narrow and the action pointed—explore the pay rates for employees in two departments, pharmacy and physical therapy. In addressing specific issues related to individual departments and work groups, however, departmental action planning also involves several factors that affect every department and work group within the organization:

- Relevance
- Job scope
- Growth and change
- Perception versus reality
- Self-perception
- Timeliness
- Needs versus wants
- Group interaction

Figure 5-1. Sample Issue and Action Statement for Department-Level Planning

Critical Issue: Prevailing perception, substantiated by the survey's numerical results and significant comment, that the pay rates for pharmacists and physical therapists here at ABC Hospital are "too low" compared to the pay rates in other hospitals.

Action Mandates:

1. Wage survey to be conducted by human resources department
2. Task force of pharmacists and physical therapists to explore market wage levels
3. Review of fiscal year's budget to explore organization's latitude in increasing salaries

Relevance

The first factor is the relevance of the individual department to the organization as a whole. In other words, how does the department support the big picture? Survey analyzers note any comments relative to the way employees in specific departments feel that the organization supports them and, conversely, how those outside the department view it. Again, responses may be either positive or negative. It is the responsibility of the individual department manager or unit supervisor to determine how this data may lead to constructing an action plan that incorporates organizational support and participation.

Job Scope

Managers also discuss with individual employees how their jobs fit into their specific department or work group and the organization as a whole. (See section III of Appendix A.) The unit supervisor or department manager may use the resultant data to open up conversations with the employees or groups of employees subsequent to the survey.

Growth and Change

All departments in a health care organization are affected by growth and change, sometimes positively and sometimes negatively. Therefore, many items on the survey address attitudes toward growth and change. Many comments and suggestions gathered in the course of the survey indicate employee reactions to proposed or actual growth in the facility (for example, new construction or expansion of services).

Although these factors certainly affect the whole organization, an individual is more likely to comment on growth–change dynamics as they affect his or her department and specific job. For example, the construction of a new ambulatory care facility on the campus of a community hospital might seem to be irrelevant to the work life of a food service employee until the employee considers the impact on his or her particular job of the additional customers brought in by the new facility.

Perception versus Reality

Another important factor in departmental and group action planning is perception versus reality. Every group within a health care organization has a specific perception of its function and personality. Often, respondents refer to groups of individuals within the organization using a specific adjective or label. The adjective or label can be positive (such as "proactive" or "progressive") or negative (such as, "uncooperative" or "arrogant"). When labeling occurs, it is noted by the survey conduct team. These important descriptive labels can then be mentioned for discussion and amplification with employees in the postsurvey meetings. In responding to a positive label, the role of the executive manager facilitating the postsurvey meeting is easy. He or she simply mentions and reinforces the positive perception. When a label is negative, however, the executive manager (with the department manager whose department is being labeled and the human resources team) examines why this label is being used and attempts to dispel the negative perception of this department.

Two important factors come into play in the perception versus reality question. First, the label being examined is used by a variety of individuals responding to the survey. A good rule of thumb is that the same label was used by at least 10 individuals out of a 500-person sample group. Second, survey analyzers must get as much supporting data as possible about *why* a particular label is being used in reference to a specific group. Then, the executive manager who facilitates the postsurvey meeting uses the label to stimulate discussion with the general work group. In subsequent department-level meetings, the individual department manager also discusses the reason why the rest of the organization labels the department in this way.

Self-Perception

Another useful factor in departmental analysis and action planning is department self-perception. Most department members feel that their department is very important to the survival of the entire organization. Accordingly, in a typical attitude survey, many comments like these appear: "Without our department, the hospital would not be here" and "Our department is the hub of the entire operation." Such comments promote an elitist attitude among certain department employees. In some cases, such attitudes are healthy; in others they create friction with other work groups. Elitist labels can be considered positive and healthy *only* when applied to the entire organization in a manner such as, "Our hospital has the best prenatal care in Cook County." Otherwise, people become angry, resentful, and so on. Accordingly, the survey conduct team and the department managers must read between the lines and use common sense and objectivity to ensure that elitist perceptions do not threaten any department's relationship with another.

Timeliness

Another important aspect of departmental action planning is timeliness. Often, for example, individuals cite on the survey situations that occurred in the distant past. In some cases, such comments are discounted if the situation referred to no longer exists. In addition, survey comments often relate to the distant future or to potential future situations that may never come to exist. For example, many comments on a survey conducted at a hospital in an industrial area concerned employees' fears about the potential closure of a local manufacturing business. Although the employees' concerns were based purely on speculation, many were focusing on the negative effect that the closure of the large employer would have on their job security.

Managers should straightforwardly discuss with employees such comments in the department-level action planning meetings. When appropriate, managers dismiss false rumors. If such rumors trouble employees organization-wide, the executive manager who facilitates the postsurvey all-staff meetings should also dispel the rumors with facts.

Needs versus Wants

In departmental action planning, the survey conduct team and individual managers separate and address the respondents' *needs* from their *wants*. Most survey respondents mention at least one thing that they feel they need from the organization or a department leader (for example, a specific piece of equipment or more fiscal resources). The survey conduct team carefully separates what an individual actually needs to get his or her job done from what he or she might want in a perfect world. Viability and relevance are essential to making a needs determination. Once a determination has been made, the department manager constructs an action plan to present at his or her briefing meeting wherein the needs and potential ways to meet them are discussed.

Department managers must also pay special attention to any suggestions given in the survey that identify needs that, if met, would improve the department. For example, members of a radiology department might express their need for a specific form to make the transmission of radiological images more efficient and effective. As another example, pharmacy department members (as evidenced by responses from 5 employees out of a department of 15) might indicate that the operation of the walk-up window would be more efficient if the department hired a part-time receptionist to help back it up.

Group Interaction

Another important aspect of health care productivity is group interaction. In a survey individuals often explain that their effectiveness or ineffectiveness is due to the interaction of department members or other colleagues. The department manager should address interpersonal dynamics with the assistance of the human resources staff and the executive manager. Sometimes, these situations require additional surveying and other organizational development assistance. (See the analysis guides in appendix B.) Most important, however, interpersonal dynamics should not be ignored after the survey process. Disregarding problems will only result in a total lack of credibility not only in the survey project but also in the manager and the organization.

Guidelines for Department-Level Meetings

Once individual department managers have been briefed by the survey conduct team, they schedule postsurvey department-level staff meetings in which information about the survey findings related specifically to each department are communicated. The postsurvey meetings may be made part of regularly scheduled department meetings. Or, the department manager may want to schedule a meeting dedicated solely to discussion of the survey outcomes. Department managers should follow four guidelines for conducting department-level briefing meetings:

- No information should be provided in a manner threatening to individuals or groups of employees. Negative information should never be communicated in an accusatory manner.
- The confidentiality of all employees must be maintained throughout the action planning and discussion processes. No comments should be attributed to specific employees unless the employee is consulted first (even if the employee revealed his or her name on the survey information sheet). For example, an employee might make a specific constructive comment but not feel comfortable in having the entire department know where it came from. In this case, the manager would ask the employee in private before the meeting whether he or she objects to having the comment attributed to him or her directly.
- All the comments and suggestions should be discussed in a positive manner, including any negative comments or specific suggestions for correcting a potentially harmful situation. The comments should be reviewed objectively, with the manager taking the lead by presenting his or her own potential solutions. The manager should also request employees to provide solutions of their own.
- The meeting should be conducted in a participative and open-ended style. Many managers have found the strategy of presenting a top 10 or top 20 list to be helpful. That is, they identify 10 or 20 specific suggestions, situations, or comments from the survey data that they feel are appropriate and beneficial for the entire department to discuss. With this approach, the emphasis is placed on discussing outcomes in a nonthreatening, productive manner.

Environmental Action Planning

In action planning for long-term change, several items on the survey explore the operational environment of the health care organization, including the current status of customer relations. As always, insights provided by the respondents are incorporated into organizational and departmental action plans. In addition, many managers, if not all of the management staff, themselves responded to the survey, and their responses constitute an effective environmental analysis.

To begin, any customer/patient insights are recorded by the survey conduct team and then reviewed by the executive management group. In almost every health care survey that the author has conducted over the past 15 years, comments about customer relations have dominated the responses from all segments of the organization. Because the needs of the customer/patient drive the operation of the health care organization, every member of the organization is fully aware of the importance of customer relations.

Analysis of Customer-Related Information

The survey conduct team takes special note of customer/patient-related feedback in the following areas:

- Negative comments made by customer/patients to employees that may provide insight into the reasons behind their dissatisfaction
- Positive comments made by customer/patients to employees that may provide direction for future service improvements
- Suggestions made by customer/patients to respondents that may help increase the efficiency and effectiveness of the health care organization as a whole
- Comments made to employees in the community, on an informal basis, that may reveal the community's perception of the health care organization
- Ideas and suggestions provided by customer/patients who are neighbors of respondents or members of their clientele within the health care organization that may prove meaningful to future action planning
- Specific comments or suggestions made by customer/patients to respondents that may be beneficial in increasing the effectiveness of specific departments, procedures, or employees

The customer/patient-related responses may also reveal valuable demographic information. For example, in many surveys the author has recently conducted, respondents have provided insight into the need for, and the practicality of, establishing women's health care units, prenatal care units, teen drug awareness programs, and an assortment of programs addressing other contemporary health care issues. In this manner, the survey may prove an effective tool in helping the organization tailor its services to emerging community needs.

Furthermore, knowledge of this type of information can prove invaluable to health care organization executives as they try to develop strategic plans and make determinations on placing priorities for the coming years. Most individuals who utilize a health care facility do not take the time to fill out a survey, infocard, or other type of customer/patient feedback mechanism. However, they will take every opportunity to relay their perceptions and ideas to neighbors who are members of the health care organization, to nurses who are attending their cases, or to receptionists who help them fill out their insurance information forms.

Analysis of Strategic Information about Customer Relations

The executive management team looks at all comments related to the customer/patient environment and identifies information pertinent to three basic areas:

- Community demands and concerns
- Community perceptions of the health care organization
- Significant changes in the health care environment

By looking at these three dynamics (discussed in more detail in the following subsections), the executive management team is able to develop a plan that addresses concerns revealed by the survey, to present the action plan for further development, and to validate existing strategic plans.

Because most managers and employees in a health care organization are also members of the community, they can provide a wealth of information about the institution as perceived by their friends, families, and neighbors. To be useful, however, this information is separated into two categories— *primary* and *secondary*. Primary data include specific experiences that the respondents shared with customer/patients or that they have had personally as customer/patients at the hospital. Secondary information includes any information survey respondents heard secondhand rather than observed or experienced directly. For example, a respondent may have been told by a customer/patient about a particular situation or given a suggestion by a former customer/patient. Primary information is often more specific in nature but can be more subjective. Secondary information, though less specific, may be more objective in that the employee has thought about it and then evaluated it in an unbiased manner. In both cases, the information can prove useful, as long as it is logically and sensibly reviewed by the survey conduct team and appropriate members of the organization's management.

Community Demands and Concerns

In analysis of strategic information about customer relations, community concerns are important considerations. Often in the past when a health care organization provided high-quality service to a community over a period of years, that community may have taken the health care provider for granted, thereby having had no particular reason or motivation to make a conscious evaluation of the quality of health care they have received. Because of increasing cost and access problems in health care, this situation has changed over the past 10 years. Today, virtually everyone has some opinion about health care services and providers. Therefore, it is vital for the survey instrument to examine customer/patient perceptions, with the goal of identifying the concerns of the community the organization serves. For example, many individuals in the community may be concerned that the organization is not growing or that it is growing too fast.

In addition, many comments may be made about the technology of health care. For example, in an attitude survey conducted at one small rural hospital, many respondents provided information from their friends and neighbors throughout the community that the hospital was inefficient in meeting their needs because it did not have an "MRI machine." Apparently, these individuals had seen several programs on television touting the benefits of MRI technology. Therefore, their expectation was that any good hospital would have one. Because their hospital did not have an MRI, they felt that they were being insufficiently served by the institution. This revelation caused a considerable degree of consternation among members of the executive group, but it also gave them a good opportunity to respond to the community concern through solid organization–community communication as well as to make provisions with a neighboring hospital to utilize its MRI equipment.

Community Perceptions of the Health Care Organization

Most individuals within the community will let their friends and neighbors at the health care facility know whether they approve of the conduct of the health care organization. Again, it is vital to understand community concerns as they relate to the environment in which the health care organization operates.

Significant Changes in the Health Care Environment

One of the current debates throughout North America concerns the public's perception of the local health care provider as a public service rather than a profit-making business. Managers in a health care setting who respond to a survey are usually more aware of the business dynamics of the health care institution and whether the community perceives the organization as a business or as a public service. However, staff employees also receive information from their friends and neighbors about the cost of health care services and the business policies of the hospital or health care provider. Therefore, it is vital for the survey conduct team to review the responses of both groups when doing environmental action planning.

Individual Employee Action Planning

Another category of survey data to be incorporated into a solid action plan for long-term change is action that can be taken by individual employees. In reviewing employee action plans, the survey conduct team must identify the following types of information:

- Prevailing attitudes held by a majority of employees organizationwide
- Prevailing attitudes held by specific groups of employees within technical groups

- Actions suggested by employees that may benefit the organization as a whole
- Actions suggested by the employees that may support the development and progress of a specific department
- Actions suggested by the employees that may help correct specific problems within their work areas
- Needs and requirements expressed by the employees that may help them perform their jobs more effectively
- Suggestions for the organization to make the work lives of its employees more productive and the workplace more progressive

These seven areas are the fundamental components of action planning for individual employees. Because managers and supervisors are also employees, their input is noted by the survey conduct team and incorporated into a comprehensive action plan for the entire organization. Furthermore, the input of managers is essential to achieving a balanced and complete organizational perspective. That is, managers often have many perceptions that are similar to those of other employees but hold other perceptions that might counterbalance perceptions held by employees who might be nonplayers or chronic complainers by nature. It is essential that the survey conduct team and senior management group obtain a full, unbiased perspective on prevailing attitudes.

Analysis of Information Pertinent to Individual Employees

When the survey conduct team and the executive management group conduct individual employee action planning, the following issues arising in survey feedback are useful to focus on:

- General concerns
- Technical resources
- Effective management
- Participatory management
- Ethics and values
- Quality improvement
- Educational opportunities
- Interpersonal relationships
- Perceptions of the organization as a whole
- Recruitment information

General Concerns
There are many areas of general employee life that respondents may bring up in an attitude survey. The survey conduct team and executive management should seriously consider employees' suggestions and comments about parking facilities, cafeteria services, and similar areas of work life.

The wage and compensation issue is always principal among these concerns. The survey team and management must be diligent in reviewing any complaints about the wage and compensation system. However, they must balance the complaints with the knowledge that most employees are not completely satisfied with their pay scale, no matter how fair or how equitable it may be in relation to current wage statistics and regional standards.

Technical Resources

Many employees use the attitude survey (especially section III) to report their needs for improved or additional technical resources. They might list, for example, equipment, changes in procedures, and/or additional resources needed to make their jobs more efficient. In fact, there might also be a common response from a group of employees about the technical needs in their area. The survey conduct team notes these types of comments and relays them directly to the department manager.

Effective Management

On attitude surveys employees often compare their notions of an ideal manager with their perceptions of their current managers or supervisors. Accordingly, the survey conduct team notes any comments relative to the effectiveness of department or unit management registered by individual employees, a group of similar employees, or members of the same department. As always, significant data and comments, both positive and negative, are recorded. The survey conduct team then provides such information to the manager in question as well as to the manager's superior.

This strategy is followed any time an employee cites a specific management problem. For example, if an employee respondent indicated that he or she perceives that a manager is "playing favorites" among individuals in a department, the situation should be evaluated by the specific manager, his or her supervisor, and the survey conduct team. In addition, the particular employee, if he or she identified himself or herself on the survey's information sheet, could be asked to speak with the manager and the manager's supervisor. This would allow the employee to explain the specific problems in more detail in a fair atmosphere.

Participatory Management

Employees often register concerns about their opportunities to participate in the management process. Particularly in the current health care era of continuous quality improvement (CQI) programs and other employee participation mechanisms, employees are encouraged to make suggestions and provide input to discussions of productivity improvement and other programs. In the attitude survey, a participative exercise in and of itself, employees are provided many opportunities to offer suggestions for improving their work lives. When appropriate, opportunities to participate in decision making and to make suggestions that may directly affect the direction of work and the accomplishment of organizational objectives are incorporated into the action plan.

Ethics and Values

An important dynamic in any health care organization involves ethical action and value-driven performance. As both individuals and group members, employees provide insight into how they feel about the organization's ethical and value systems. The survey conduct team records for discussion in postsurvey all-staff meetings any employee comments about the organization as an ethical health care provider. Any specific allegations of unethical behavior or non-value-driven performance are also recorded for subsequent discussion. Employees may observe breaches of ethical performance firsthand. Therefore, they are excellent resources in not only identifying problems but, more important, in providing solutions. For example, many employees fully understand their organization's stated mission and values. Every day, they compare actions observed with the tenets expressed in the organization's mission and value statements. When there is disparity, they recognize it immediately.

When survey data suggest that disparities exist, a good strategy for the manager conducting the postsurvey meeting is to present the value statement and ask for specific examples of lapses. In utilizing this strategy, the discussion becomes nonthreatening while preserving the respondent's confidentiality. At the same time, it accomplishes the goal of addressing perceived ethical problems.

Quality Improvement

Because quality is the most important aspect of health care, many employees naturally offer suggestions on how quality could be improved. Usually, employees make suggestions related to their individual job roles. Many employees know what they need to perform their jobs at the highest possible level of quality and efficiency; they also know what barriers exist to prevent them from doing so. Accordingly, the survey conduct team notes any quality improvement suggestions and makes them components of the emerging action plan.

Educational Opportunities

Education is an important component in any successful health care organization. The attitude survey provides employees the opportunity to suggest what kind of training they require to become more proficient in their jobs. The survey conduct team tries to record comments verbatim and incorporate them into the action plan. The comments are recorded verbatim so that their meaning will be fully and accurately conveyed. (Additionally, certain terms and phrases might be familiar to the managers in particular departments. These managers can then assess the terms' specific meanings.) In doing so, the survey conduct team gives the executive reviewing manager facilitating the postsurvey meetings the opportunity to discuss training and development more specifically and practically with the employees who attend the meetings. The survey is, therefore, the first step of a needs analysis relative to organizational strategic planning for staff training and development.

Interpersonal Relationships

Individual employee perspectives of interpersonal relationships usually appear somewhere in the survey's suggestions and comments sections. Some employees use the survey as an opportunity to laud the contribution or work approach of specific colleagues; others to vilify fellow employees. In both cases, the survey conduct team notes the specific comments. Then, with the employees' managers, they develop an action plan for reinforcing positive relationships and resolving any problems. It is important for the manager and the survey conduct team to try to determine *why* the employees in one department seem to be working well together while another department's employees are caught up in ongoing conflict. The intervention of the human resources department, particularly its employee relations specialists, should be requested as needed.

Perceptions of the Organization as a Whole

Survey results may also reveal employees' perceptions of the organization as a whole and its future. Together, these perceptions represent an estimate of the staff's overall level of motivation and allegiance. Employees are likely to be loyal to an organization that is growing positively, demonstrates a sense of allegiance to its employees, and provides opportunities for employee growth and development. Therefore, survey results from this area can reveal a lot about the current state and future health of the organization.

Recruitment Information

An often-overlooked area for employee action planning is recruitment. In many cases, employees know the technical requirements of specific jobs better than the managers who supervise them. Viable information on recruitment strategies provided by employees should be utilized by the organization in action planning. Additionally, employees are encouraged to provide information on what recruitment standards should be and where certain professionals can be recruited.

Developing and Communicating the Organization's Action Plan

Once the analysis of the survey results is complete and departmental, environmental, and individual action plans developed, it is time for the survey conduct team to help executive management develop the organization's over-all action plan. This action plan defines the organization's overall objectives, plans for action, and specific responses to issues revealed by the survey results.

When the survey conduct team and the executive management group consider the development and distribution of the organization's action plan, they should meet, regardless of the format or the timing or the action plan itself, six important requirements:

1. The action plan must be clear-cut.
2. The action plan must encourage maximum participation from all members of the organization.
3. The action plan must focus on the organization's objectives.
4. The action plan must be tied as closely as possible to the results of the survey.
5. The action plan must be comprehensive in scope and specific in terms of objectives but relatively general in terms of specific dynamics in order to encourage maximum participation among all members of the organization.
6. The action plan must not promise miracles, but it should promise significant action.

Development of the Written Action Plan

The written action plan should include all of the results of the survey, beginning with the numerical data. As illustrated in figure 5-2, the overall action plan includes four sections: a tabulation of the numerical results, a list of the respondents' comments and suggestions, a list of critical issues, and the specific plans for action.

Figure 5-2. Key Elements of the Action Plan

Numerical Results	Comments and Suggestions
• Response rate • Percentages • "Shadings"	• Collated • Organizationally pertinent • Significant
Critical Issues	Plans for Action
• Clarity • Substantiation • Relevance	• Definitive • Progressive • Participative

Numerical Results

The basic numerical tabulation displays all of the quantitative results of the survey. Inclusion of these tabulations underscores credibility and straight-forwardness to the written action plan.

Comments and Suggestions

The action plan also reports all significant respondent comments and suggestions selected for inclusion by the survey conduct team. These comments and suggestions for action must be accepted by the executive management team as viable, relevant, and applicable to the organization's objectives. The number of comments and suggestions in the written action plan should not total more than 20 for any organization of 500 or more. This number represents a norm within the organization. That is, a certain percentage of individuals throughout the organization have registered these suggestions and comments.

However, when suggestions or comments offered by one individual or a small group of individuals have merit, they should also be listed in the action plan. Such suggestions and comments might include any of the following:

- Outstanding suggestions that the organization can implement immediately with clear, positive effect
- Citations of excellent performance by an individual member of the organization or by a particular department
- Comments or suggestions that merit discussion among individual employee groups

Critical Issues

The overall action plan includes a list of critical issues. There should be about 10 critical issues addressed that are essential to employees and managers alike and represent the basic areas essential to the organization's success. (Figure 5-1 illustrated a description of a critical issue and the presentation of this issue within the context of an action plan.)

The critical issues are distilled in the action plan by utilizing several methods. First, significant issues that were registered in the survey's "strongly agree," "agree," "neutral," "disagree," and "strongly disagree" response categories in the survey (as detailed in the analysis guides in appendix B) should be listed. For example, if communication were shown to be a pressing issue as evidenced by high percentages of strong agreement or strong disagreement in the survey, it would merit critical issue status in the action plan.

Second, any issue that is considered particularly timely should be included. For example, due to nationwide reform initiatives, most health care organizations are currently undergoing an extraordinary amount of change. Therefore, reaction to change in the organization might be a significant issue. As another example, if an organization recently underwent a bid for unionization, employee relations would become a critical issue.

Plans for Action

The action plan contains descriptions of the actions the organization plans to undertake in the near future. These actions should be closely tied to input from the survey. For example, organizations have used a simple two-part process (see figure 5-3) whereby a perception or conclusion from the survey is listed and the action to be taken in response. This clear-cut approach encourages employees to make additional suggestions and provide further input in addressing a particular issue. That is, due to the specific nature of the presentation, employees clearly understand the focus of the discussion and feel confident that they can provide suggestions and input without fear of reprisal. Other organizations have used lists of the top 10 or 20 actions to be taken. Both strategies demonstrate to respondents that their input is valued and that the organization is setting a plan of action for improving effectiveness and productivity.

Other organizations have tried more novel approaches. For example, some have designated several actions (perhaps five) that the organization deems to be significant. These actions might include, for example, "the creation of an employee task force on _____" or "the conduct of a wage survey to determine whether wages are fair and equitable." Because the implementation and detailed execution of these actions is not fully established prior to the presentation of the action plan, the employees have the opportunity to provide additional input on both.

Distribution of the Written Action Plan

Once the action plan is developed and written, it is distributed. The timing of publication for the action plan depends on several factors, including the following:

- How large is the organization?
- Is the organization currently dealing with any crisis situations?

Figure 5-3. Two-Part Approach to Action Plan Presentation

Perception/Conclusion: Most employees do not know what the five-year strategic plan for the organization contains relative to growth and basic objectives

Action Plan: Distribution of plan overview with next monthly employee newsletter

- Is the general attitude of the employees overtly negative?
- Do employees have any preconceived ideas about the survey results?
- Have rumors about the survey outcomes been circulating?
- What is the normal level of employee participation?
- How much interest in survey results has been generated?

Many organizations find it useful to publish and distribute the action plan prior to the postsurvey meetings. This allows employees an opportunity to review all survey results and the proposed action plan, thereby fine-tuning their comments for the postsurvey meetings. Other organizations distribute the action plans during the postsurvey meetings. This method allows employees an opportunity to look at the material with a fresh eye as it is being presented. It also gives the meeting leaders the opportunity to answer any employee questions about the survey quickly and personally.

Some organizations distribute the action plan after the all-staff meetings, using the meetings as opportunities to continue development of the action plan with direct employee participation. For example, meeting leaders might present the survey outcomes or conclusions and then ask the employees attending the sessions to develop a set of action plans. This approach works well in small organizations, but it can be difficult to manage in large organizations. One drawback of this approach may be that employees respond in a very broad fashion rather than focusing on action plans for addressing specific issues.

Another strategy is for the survey conduct team and executive management to publish a preliminary action plan, then conduct the all-staff postsurvey meetings, and finally produce a "final" action plan based on the reactions and contributions of employees at the meetings. This strategy allows optimum opportunity for participation by all members of the organization, as well as providing a focus for discussions throughout the survey process. Another benefit of this strategy is that a more specific action plan can be formulated (as demonstrated in the case study reported in chapter 6).

Conducting Postsurvey All-Staff Meetings

Usually, the last phase of the survey process is conducting the postsurvey informational meetings for all employees and managers. In this meeting or series of meetings, all the results of the survey, as well as the action plan that the organization has established by the combined efforts of the survey conduct team and senior management, are explained in detail and freely discussed. Publication of the action plan before, during, or after the presentation is an important component of the survey process.

Scheduling and Notification of the Meetings

The conduct of the action plan presentation is extremely important. To encourage the participation of all of the organization members, the post-survey meetings should be scheduled within a month of the survey's conclusion and conducted several times in order to allow all members of the organization the opportunity to participate.

Notification of the action plan presentation should be given at least two weeks prior to the actual sessions. All sessions should be held within a week's time, usually in a Wednesday-to-Wednesday span. This allows most individuals on vacation to attend a meeting without changing their plans. The meetings should also be scheduled at various times of the day to allow night-shift, day-shift, and part-time employees to attend.

The meetings should be held in common, accessible areas (conference rooms and cafeterias, for example). Although, there is no magic number for the number of participants who show up at any meeting, usually, a maximum of 40 individuals is considered to be workable. More than 40 individuals make reticent employees even less inclined to speak in front of a large group.

The sessions can be scheduled in either a random or a controlled fashion. Sign-up sheets can be distributed throughout the organization and employees allowed to sign up and attend as desired. Or, given the operational requirements of certain departments, department managers may schedule employees for particular meetings, in order not to disrupt operations. Either type of scheduling is acceptable. However, there can be no appearance that games are being played relative to employees attending the briefing sessions.

Some organizations allow only managers to attend the action plan presentations. This restriction, more common in health care organizations of more than 1,000 employees, is due simply to lack of time. That is, there is not enough time for each and every employee to attend a briefing session. If an organization decides to use this strategy, it is imperative that individual managers are given instructions on how to present the action plan to their department members and staff employees. It is the responsibility of the survey conduct team and the hospital's education department to ensure that all managers know how to present the survey results to employees as well as gather employee information and specific comments on the results. This strategy can be risky because some employees may not be as open and forthcoming to their supervising manager as they might be in a general forum. Organization leaders must use common sense and knowledge of their organization in deciding what type and who to schedule for action plan presentation meetings.

Meeting Format

The postsurvey meetings should be conducted by the executive manager of the organization (usually the CEO) or another member of senior management.

A member of the survey conduct team should assist the senior manager with the presentation to help answer specific questions or discuss particular segments of the survey. The meetings should be about two hours in length, the first part dedicated to a straightforward review of the survey results followed by the conclusions, and, finally, presentation of the action plan. As previously discussed in this chapter, all four parts of the overall action plan — numerical results, comments and suggestions, critical issues, and action plans — should be included in the presentation.

Presentation should be very straightforward and on the level. There should be no illusion that games are being played with the data or other elements of the survey. Therefore, the author suggests that meeting facilitators use visual aids in presenting survey results. These visual aids, usually overheads showing the numerical results, can be augmented by handouts distributed to each employee, either as part of the action plan publication or in loose-leaf pages. The survey numbers should be presented clearly, utilizing a shading technique to highlight percentages (see figure 5-4).

The individuals conducting the meeting should emphasize the positive outcomes, for example including any responses citing where the organization is doing a particularly good job. However, the meeting facilitators should present any negative issues raised by the survey clearly and give all meeting participants the opportunity to discuss why such a negative situation exists and, more important, to make suggestions toward solution. Any proposed management solutions to negative situations should also be presented forthrightly and directly in the meeting.

Following presentation of the four segments of the action plan, ample opportunity should be provided for individuals to make comments and suggestions while the information presented is still fresh in their minds. This comments and suggestions session serves as a transition to the second hour of the action planning presentation, which is completely respondent generated. In this open forum, participants should be able to ask any and all

Figure 5-4. Shading Technique Using Blue

SA	A	N	D	SD
28%	32%	11%	18%	11%
royal blue	navy blue	teal	medium blue	teal

SA = Strongly Agree
A = Agree
N = Neutral
D = Disagree
SD = Strongly Disagree

questions they might have relative to the survey. At the same time, the facilitator should try to get a firm understanding of the rationale behind the participants' comments.

While the facilitator conducts the second half of the session, the individual from the survey conduct team makes copious notes of the participants' comments and suggestions. Any overtly negative statements should be managed properly by the facilitator. For example, if an individual said, "I have a problem with _____," the facilitator should immediately ask for a solution to the problem. If an individual gave a particularly negative "speech" during the second hour, the facilitator must take the responsibility to ask the individual for a solution to the problem, rather than to encourage him or her to make a speech redefining a problem that has already been established.

In the second part of the meeting, the individual conducting the presentation also can validate various perceptions raised. As comments and suggestions are offered, the facilitator can ask the assembly such questions as, "Is this real?" or "Do you buy this?" Some respondents will be more active in the presentational process than they were in the survey. They feel more comfortable discussing things verbally than on paper. However, those individuals who feel more comfortable with confidentiality and a written instrument, should not be put on the spot by the facilitator.

Finally, at the conclusion of the second hour of the presentation, the facilitator should ask meeting attendees five questions:

1. Is there anything else you wish to discuss?
2. Are we headed in the right direction?
3. What other solutions should we consider?
4. Is the survey basically accurate?
5. Did we miss anything in the survey process?

By asking these questions, the presentation facilitator ensures that maximum employee contribution has been achieved, and an optimum amount of data generated. Now, it is time for the organization's senior management to incorporate all viable comments and suggestions into the final action plan. As illustrated in the case study in chapter 6, this entire survey process can be of major benefit to a health care organization and well worth its time and effort.

Implementing the Organization's Action Plan

Implementation of action plans is an enormous topic, and this book's focus is on *conducting* an organizational survey. However, the case study in chapter 6 illustrates an organization's implementation of an action plan. Additionally,

Lombardi's *Progressive Health Care Management Strategies* (Chicago: American Hospital Publishing, 1992) addresses this issue in more depth.

Conclusion

After survey results have been analyzed, action planning is undertaken utilizing survey response data. This chapter discussed planning for immediate action, planning for long-term change, and departmental action planning, all necessary components for completing a successful attitude survey.

Chapter 6 ==

Case Study: Avalon Park Hospital

Introduction

The following case study, based on the author's actual consulting experience, is a composite of the actions taken by several hospitals. This case study illustrates the entire survey process in a health care organization. Many aspects of this case study provide realistic examples of material previously detailed in the text. Additionally, new approaches and ideas will be offered.

Avalon Park Hospital, founded in 1946, is a midsize community hospital located in the Purple Mountain region of eastern Pennsylvania. The hospital, a not-for-profit facility, employs approximately 1,000 employees in a service area encompassing a 50-mile radius.

The Purple Mountain region is noted for two main industries—tourism and transportation and distribution. The Purple Mountains are a tourist destination featuring a variety of ski resorts; summertime attractions; lakes and rivers; and an impressive roster of hotels and resorts. Therefore, the area is well populated year round.

The area is also a transportation and distribution hub for the entire eastern United States. In the early part of the century, the area was a well-known railroad center with over a dozen railroads transporting freight and passengers from the midwest and other parts of the United States to New York, Philadelphia, and other large eastern cities. After the decline of the railroad, the trucking distribution industry utilized many of the terminals and other facilities left behind by the railroad industry. The Purple Mountain region had never really had a period of sustained economic decline until recently, when the area suffered a minor economic recession due to the decline of several manufacturing firms and other businesses.

Because of the minor economic recession, Avalon Park Hospital has undergone several changes in recent years. First, it absorbed Shileen Memorial, a smaller community hospital, approximately 30 miles from Avalon Park Hospital. This hospital, during its peak in the late 1960s, employed approximately

300 employees. However, because of declining revenue and other environmental circumstances, it was absorbed three years ago by the larger Avalon Park Hospital. The merged organization's name became Avalon Park/Shileen Health Facility.

Another economic dynamic affecting Avalon Park Hospital is the emergence of the Purple Mountain HMO Program. This health maintenance organization utilizes for its vast membership many of Avalon Park's physicians and services. The HMO's membership extends to workers at the hotels, the resorts, and many of the distribution companies in the region. The HMO figures prominently in the financial prosperity of Avalon Park Hospital, as well as the Shileen Health Facility.

Furthermore, four years ago, Avalon Park Hospital established an outpatient clinic for many of the distribution workers, managers, and hotel personnel. This clinic is located in the major town of Bridgewater, approximately four miles from the Avalon Park main facility in the city of Avalon Park.

Two years ago, the Avalon Park management group also absorbed the Mountain Home for the Aging, a smaller facility employing 200. The reason for this takeover was again the declining economic prosperity of the overall region. It was also due to the fact that the HMO group felt that it was in the hospital's best interest to absorb a home for the aging because such a facility would help bring medical services to the retired members of the local community more comprehensively. Because many of the retirees of the Purple Mountain area are now members of the HMO group, it was imperative for the hospital to make this strategic business move.

With all these changes, Avalon Park Hospital currently has an overall employee base of approximately 1,500 individuals, with 500 working in facilities other than the main hospital. All employees, however, are still administered by a central human resources department, that operates under the aegis of the Avalon Park Hospital executive management team. The hospital has been relatively profitable in recent years thanks to the emergent HMO and favorable conditions in the Avalon Park metropolitan area. The city of Avalon Park (population approximately 35,000) has been growing due to the relocation of a major distribution company, Marina Distribution, from Louisiana to the Avalon Park area. This relocation brought over 1,000 new jobs to the area and increased the number of HMO members and potential Avalon Park Hospital customer/patients.

The Organization

Avalon Park Hospital has been fortunate to have undergone little turnover among its executive management team. Fred Fabian, the chief executive officer (CEO), has headed the hospital for 11 years. A relatively progressive administrator, he was the main catalyst in the absorption of the Mountain

Home for the Aging and Shileen Memorial into the Avalon Park Hospital organization. Previous to being CEO, Fabian was the director of human resources for Avalon Park Hospital and prides himself on "knowing his people" and ensuring that the hospital enforces its corporate slogan, "We put people first in everything we do."

The hospital's chief operating officer (COO) is Monica Cirello. With the hospital for approximately 18 years, Cirello started as a staff nurse and worked her way through the ranks of nursing management and into the main operations position. Like Fabian, she believes that Avalon Park Hospital does an extraordinary job in terms of "making the human touch the hospital's best product."

Reporting to Monica Cirello is the director of nursing, Shelly Tyrone. Tyrone's responsibilities include managing the facility's largest employee segment—approximately 450 nurses.

Caitlin Prescott is the hospital's chief financial officer (CFO). She is also the most junior member of the executive management team, both in years with the organization (five) and chronologically. Prior to her arrival at Avalon Park Hospital, Prescott was a financial director for a smaller distribution company in the Purple Mountain area. She learned about the business of health care largely on the job, first as the budget director for the hospital and then as the accounting director. Prescott assumed the responsibilities of CFO two years ago with the retirement of the previous CFO.

Rick Colina is the chief administrative officer of the hospital. The director of security, the director of personnel, the director of employee education, the director of food services, and several other administrative positions all report to Colina.

Kirk Fremont, the director of human resources, has been with the hospital for the same amount of time as Colina, over nine years. It was Colina who first hired Fremont as the hospital's associate personnel director, and these two individuals carry out their jobs in a partnerlike manner. (See figure 6-1, the organizational chart.)

At the suggestion of board member Marina Clark (of the Marina Distribution Company family), the health care organization's management is currently considering a name change for the institution. This name change would be more inclusive of the smaller entities recently absorbed by the hospital. The new name also would highlight the progressive nature of the overall organization, such as the emergence of the HMO. Organization management is considering conducting a survey to select a new name for the merged organization. The survey will be done from a marketing perspective and seek to select a more accurately representative name for the "new" organization.

The organization's reputation seems in accordance with its value statement (presented to all employees and posted throughout the entire organization). See figure 6-2. Furthermore, little dissatisfaction has been voiced by the organization's employees. Although executive management is currently

**Figure 6-1. Organization Chart, Avalon Park
Hospital Corporation**

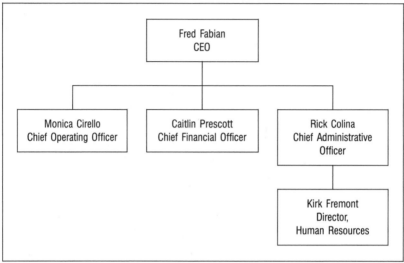

Figure 6-2. Avalon Park Value Statement

- The customer/patient is the most important member of our organization.
- Taking care of people means taking care of *our* people.
- Dignity and compassion are our two main products.
- We will use all available technology and talent to assist those in need.
- We are a community-based public trust in the truest sense of the phrase.

satisfied with the organization's position in the community and its reputation with its customer/patients, they are concerned about the organization appearing to be too large or growing too fast. And despite the overall positive nature of the current organization, the executive management team does have some concerns:

1. Potential interest in unionization among nurses (due to rising national trends in this area)
2. Complete absorption and affiliation of employees in the clinics, the Home for the Aging, and the Shileen facility, all of whose employees have always seen themselves as being "different" from Avalon Park employees
3. Underlying employee resentment and potential dissatisfaction with several human resources programs and with employee life in the Avalon Park organization in general
4. Employee concerns about the future and positive growth of the organization, paralleling the economic recession of the general area (with the

exception of the Marina Distribution Company relocation from Louisiana, there have been few economic bright spots in the Purple Mountain region)

The last concern is the most potentially troubling for Avalon Park employees. Many individuals who work at the hospital are long-term employees and the majority of them were born and raised in the Purple Mountain area or nearby. Many of the employees' families and friends work in the resorts and those resorts received a blow when the state legislature failed to ratify an amendment approving legalized casino gambling. This failed amendment, coupled with the state legislature's blocking the construction of a major highway to the area, has crippled the financial prosperity of several of the well-known and long-established hotel resorts.

Knowing the economic problems of the employee population of a health care organization reflect regional economic problems, Avalon Park Hospital's executive management group decided to conduct an attitude survey for all employees. The survey's objectives were to verify whether the four assumptions previously presented were, indeed, legitimate reasons for management concern. Additionally, the organization was interested in employee perception of management, job content, the organization as a whole, as well as other general issues important to the organization's progress. Because the hospital lacked a strong suggestion system in the past, it was hoped that the attitude survey would offer employees the opportunity to make comments and suggestions that might be useful in redefining the hospital's actions, goals, and strategic imperatives.

Six years ago, a needs-analysis survey was conducted to identify topics for employee and manager training and development. However, no attitude survey had ever been done at Avalon Park Hospital. And since the needs analysis was conducted, the organization has implemented few human resources innovations. Due to the organization's rapid growth, Kirk Fremont and his staff centered their efforts on simply trying to hire enough individuals to staff the new clinic, as well as to take the necessary actions to assimilate all of the Home for the Aging and the Shileen employees. Fremont and his staff had little time for such "extra" work as employee attitude surveys. However, because of its concern for employee welfare and desire to receive optimum employee input at this particular time, its executive management felt that an employee attitude survey had become a pressing need.

Because of operational budget limitations, Fremont decided to utilize the survey instrument and process contained in this text as the basis for his survey. To assist him in the process, he hired Dr. Beavis Anderson, a local college professor, to help distribute the survey and act as a neutral third party in analyzing the results and making the employee presentations.

Preparation of the Survey

Fremont asked to make a presentation at the executive management meeting. At this meeting, CEO Fabian and his entire staff took the opportunity to review all the items to be used in the survey. They decided that by using all of the items in appendix A of this book, they would receive a comprehensive view of their organization. However, under the heading of general issues in section IV, three new items more pertinent to their particular facility were substituted for those in the survey text. (See figure 6-3.)

At this initial meeting, the executive management team also decided on five definitive survey objectives they hoped to achieve:

1. To get a general sense of prevailing employee and manager attitudes toward the organization
2. To gather as many employee comments and suggestions as possible in one sweeping effort
3. To determine whether executive management's four major concerns about the employee population are valid
4. To offer employees the opportunity to make suggestions about the organization's progress and innovation
5. To ensure that all employees—including those at the three "new" facilities—are provided an equal opportunity to offer input to their new organization in the interest of making a stronger whole

In order to achieve these objectives, Fremont, with the help of Professor Anderson, decided to establish a three-month time line for the survey process. First, they planned to establish a survey conduct team composed of managers and employees to assist in survey distribution and collection. Second, Fremont and Anderson decided it would take approximately one month to print the surveys, one month to distribute and collect them, and another month for the team (in concert with executive management) to analyze the results and develop action plans. Therefore, on September 1, the date this initial meeting was held, the executive management team made a commitment to assist Fremont in bringing the survey process to completion by December 1. This time frame was excellent because survey results and related action plans would be established by the end of the year and prior to the busy holiday season in the Purple Mountains. This time line helped provide impetus for employees and managers to begin the new year on a positive note.

Figure 6-3. New Section IV Questions Based on Appendix A

1. I feel that the people who work at Shileen and the Home for the Aging are "full partners" in the Avalon Park organization.
2. All of the facilities in the Avalon Park organization are considered "good places to work at" by most members of our community.
3. I feel, for the most part, that our organization is growing "in the right way" and "at the right pace."

The executive management team made the decision to let Fremont be in charge of creating the survey conduct team. The only provision the executive management team made was that along with Professor Anderson and Kirk Fremont, four managers and eight employees (four from the Avalon Park facility, one from the Mountain Home for the Aging, one from the Shileen facility, and one from the clinic) serve on the survey conduct team. The final employee representative was Natalie Pine, a compensation clerk who works in the human resources area. She was selected because of her long tenure with the organization and her reputation as a positive presence among the employee population. The survey conduct team planned to begin work within the next two weeks. There was to be an initial meeting to help prepare the printing of the survey and to compose letters to all organization members regarding the upcoming survey distribution.

Fred Fabian drafted a letter to all employees in which he alerted them that a survey would be distributed on October 1 and encouraged their participation in the survey process. Fabian asked all managers to read this letter at their September monthly department meetings and to include a copy of the letter with employees' paychecks. This letter also assured employees of survey confidentiality and promised to provide in December a series of presentational meetings and action plans based on the survey results. This letter was also posted on several bulletin boards throughout all organization facilities and distributed in the cafeterias and coffee rooms utilized by night-shift employees. By the end of September, employees at all four Avalon Park organization locations had been made aware of the survey.

The survey conduct team then undertook the preparation of the survey for publication. The survey conduct team decided to attempt to make the survey instrument as cosmetically pleasing as possible. They created a booklet with a purple cover prominently featuring the suggested logo of the Avalon Park Hospital System (the suggested new name for the corporation). By putting the logo on the cover of the survey instrument, the survey conduct team hoped to discover whether it triggered a positive or negative reaction from employees.

The booklet's first page contained a letter from Fred Fabian again explaining the survey's purpose and promising confidentiality and presentation of survey results and subsequent related action plans. The next page was the administrative data page, on which employees can supply information (including name, title, shift, organization, and status, for example, part- or full-time) on an optional basis. The survey conduct team believed that many employees would be willing to fill out the entire identification page.

The survey itself followed these two pages. Each section of the survey was composed of 10 items. At the top of each page there was a set of instructions and at the bottom of each section there was ample room for comments and suggestions. The information imparted by the instructions was twofold. First, the instructions reiterated how the employees were to utilize the *strongly agree, agree, neutral, disagree,* and *strongly disagree* categories. Second, there was a sentence in the instructions describing the intent of each section (similar to the information provided in the appendix material of this text).

The final page of the survey was a general comments and suggestions page on which employees were encouraged to write any other comments and/or suggestions they felt were pertinent. The survey conduct team felt that this final page was important because the Avalon Park Hospital System was a new entity and many employees had never had the opportunity to voice any suggestions or opinions about the re-formed organization.

The survey conduct team stumbled upon an interesting dilemma. That is, the executive management team did not give them specific instructions on what to call the survey. Accordingly, the survey conduct team had to decide whether to call the process "an attitude survey," "an organizational study," or "a climate study."

The word *attitude* in the eastern United States usually has a negative connotation. That is, some individuals may say, "that person sure has a real attitude," meaning that the person is a "pain in the neck." The team, therefore, rejected the title "attitude survey," fearing that it was too confusing. Furthermore, the survey conduct team felt that using the term "attitude" might have inadvertently limited employees to providing comments strictly in regards to their "attitudes," neglecting to provide suggestions and/or new ideas for the organization.

For two reasons neither *climate survey* nor *climate study* had particular appeal for the survey group. First, the word *climate* in a resort area usually relates to the environmental climate (the weather). Second, the economic "climate" of the area was not particularly healthy at that time.

By utilizing the process of elimination, the survey conduct team decided on *organizational study.* This name encompassed the organization as a whole—including the clinic, the Home for the Aging, and the Shileen facility. Also, the term *study* underscored the fact that analysis would be conducted relative to the survey results. The survey conduct team felt that because "organizational study" was the most user-friendly title, it would encourage the most open, positive response. Accordingly, the front page of the survey instrument read "Avalon Park Healthcare System — Organizational Study."

One of the survey conduct team members was Brian McBride, the pharmacy manager. Due to the volume of the hospital's and the three outlying facilities' pharmacy activities, McBride displayed an uncanny understanding of people because he deals with many on a daily basis. McBride suggested to the survey conduct team that many managers and employees were apprehensive about the survey. These individuals felt as though it might be an undercover operation to try to identify the "bad eggs" and subsequently get rid of them. Additionally, McBride heard many comments at the outlying facilities voicing the opinion that the survey was an attempt to try to force the Avalon Park "way of doing things down the throats of the new people."

Other survey conduct team members agreed with McBride's observations. The problem then became what to do about it. In response, the survey conduct team decided to conduct several focus groups both to dispel any apprehensions about the survey and to fine-tune the survey instrument. In order to accomplish this, five focus groups of 15 individuals each were scheduled at the four facilities. One focus group was conducted during the day shift at Avalon Park Hospital and another during the night shift. Other focus groups were held during the day shift at the three facilities (although night-shift employees of these three facilities were represented).

The focus groups reviewed the survey but did not complete it. Professor Anderson conducted the test groups with the assistance of two members of the survey conduct team. The focus groups allowed the survey conduct team members to see how the survey might actually work. Survey conduct team members dutifully recorded all focus groups' reactions and comments. After conducting all five focus groups, the survey conduct team decided that four changes must be made to make the survey more effective:

1. The words *manager* and *supervisor* must be used jointly in many sentences, as employees in all four facilities utilize different terms for managers. In some cases, supervisor is a designation for someone who is acting as a manager.
2. All references to "my organization" should be changed to "our organization." This will help respondents realize that the organization is not comparing one facility to another (such as Avalon Park Hospital to Shileen).
3. The final comments and suggestions page instructions should be reinforced to give individuals ideas about what type of suggestions to make. Instead of just saying "any additional comments or suggestions," the new instructions will include "Please include on this page any further comments or suggestions about the organization, your job, or other important dimensions of your work life here at Avalon Park Healthcare System. Use additional pages if necessary."
4. An amendment will be added to Fabian's letter encouraging individuals to fill out the survey, and a sentence that made completing the survey seem a requirement of employment will be eliminated. Many of the employees who received notice about the survey in their paycheck felt as though they were mandated to complete the survey. Although a minority of employees held this view, this minority was consistent at all four organization locations. Therefore, the final sentences of Fabian's letter in the survey booklet became:

   "In order to make our system better, we need your input. While this is a voluntary process, your input is vital, and we feel everyone should have a voice as we try to build a progressive, dynamic health care system."

Having received and addressed the focus-group feedback, the survey conduct team was justly satisfied that the instrument was ready for distribution. To the best knowledge of the survey conduct team, all the organization's managers had informed their employees that the survey would be distributed during the week of October 1. The forms were then printed in cosmetically appealing purple booklets with the system's logo on the cover and were stored in a stack of boxes in Fremont's office.

Distribution and Collection of the Survey

The survey conduct team decided to use a variety of distribution processes to get the survey into the hands of the entire employee population of the Avalon Park Healthcare system. The survey conduct team encouraged manager participation by conducting four management meetings. These meetings, held in the form of luncheons, were scheduled successively from Monday through Thursday during the first week of October.

The lunches were held at Oogie's Cafe, a popular restaurant near the Avalon Park Hospital. All the organization's managers were invited to attend a luncheon on the day most convenient to their schedule. The survey conduct team initially considered having a luncheon at each one of the four facilities but decided to make the process more collective by inviting the managers to come to Oogie's Cafe for lunch. However, the managers could pick the day most convenient for them. This strategy provided the survey conduct team the primary benefit of having all manager surveys completed during the first week of October. The secondary benefit was that managers from all four facilities had the opportunity to meet each other, work together on the survey process, and provide collective feedback.

During the luncheon meetings, Fred Fabian addressed the managers for approximately 15 minutes. He discussed strategic plans for the hospital and then turned the meeting over to Kirk Fremont. Fremont explained the organization's attempt to collect employee opinions through conduction of the survey. He told the managers that not only was their participation in the survey process important, but their encouragement of employees to complete the survey was very important as well. Fremont then distributed the surveys with Professor Anderson's assistance, and, subsequent to eating lunch, all of the managers completed them. Oogie's Cafe is a relatively large facility, and to ensure their own confidentiality, many managers went outside (where there were benches) and completed the survey in private. Other managers completed the survey at their tables. Survey completion varied from 5 to 50 minutes, depending on each manager's amount of input and his or her desire to provide specific information. Fortunately, except for four members of the Shileen management staff, no managers had vacations scheduled for this week. However, the vacationing individuals made a special effort to attend the

Thursday meeting. Fabian thanked them personally for participating in the survey and encouraged them to highlight their efforts to participate as an example to their employees.

By utilizing the managers' luncheon strategy, the survey conduct team received a 100 percent response from the managers. The team then shifted its attention to distributing the survey to the employees. With the support of the board and senior management, the survey conduct team set up tables at the entrance to the employee cafeterias in all four facilities. These tables were set up during the day and night shifts on the first two successive Thursdays and Fridays in October. Employees were given an incentive to complete the survey in the form of a voucher for a free meal at the employee cafeteria during these days. Because the employee cafeteria already operates on a discounted basis, this was not a huge incentive. It was, however, a little "extra benefit" for individuals who at least picked up surveys with meal vouchers inside.

The survey conduct team members manning the tables noticed an interesting dynamic occurring during survey distribution. They mentally noted how some individuals completed the surveys immediately, while others did so on their own time utilizing other survey collection boxes set up in the facilities. The survey conduct team placed collection boxes at two other locations in each facility—the lobby and by the tables utilized for survey distribution. All collection boxes were clearly taped with only a single slot at the top through which to insert surveys. The tape assured the employees that the surveys were being handled in a confidential manner and that the boxes would not be opened until the prearranged public opening on October 14, the collection deadline.

All survey conduct team members diligently reminded employees about returning their surveys. Initially, the survey conduct team had considered the idea of providing employees an incentive for completing the survey (perhaps a raffle based on a random drawing of the survey). However, based on the focus groups' suggestions, the team decided not to resort to any devices that might be perceived as gimmicks. Collectively, the focus groups had noted that anything appearing "gimmicky" would give respondents the impression that the survey was a frivolous exercise and that the results would not be taken seriously. So, instead of using a particular collection device, the survey conduct team relied on encouragement to achieve maximum possible survey response. Fred Fabian notified all members of his executive management staff to remind their respective chain-of-command managers that the surveys were due October 14 and that all employees should participate at their own comfort level. Additionally, many survey conduct team members asked the more supportive employees to remind their peers to return the surveys.

The survey conduct team used five strategies (some previously mentioned) to ensure a maximum response rate:

1. A special section in the employee newsletter about the survey, complete with a reminder of the due date for return
2. The posting of various notices about the survey on bulletin boards in all four facilities
3. A notice placed in paycheck envelopes to remind employees to return the surveys by the 14th and to encourage, but not require, participation
4. Announcements of the survey due date by executive management team members in employee forums and other normal communication venues
5. An article in the local paper, *The Avalon Park Press,* about the survey, including the due date for return

The final strategy was unique. Because Rick Colina's sister, the local paper's editor, knew of and was interested in covering the story, mention in the paper seemed a natural strategy for publicizing the survey and thereby encouraging employees (most of whom were members of the community) to return the completed forms. Furthermore, the publicity about the survey made many employees feel less skeptical about the survey's importance. "If it was in the paper, it must be important," was one employee's comment. Additionally, many individuals in the Avalon Park area not affiliated with the health care organization were interested in the survey results, which the paper promised to publish in a later edition. Although this strategy could appear to some as overkill, it demonstrated the administration's dedication to maintaining open communication with members of its service community.

As October 14 approached, the survey conduct team distributed a final bulletin at the beginning of each shift in all four facilities. The bulletin encouraged employees to return the survey by October 14 and also informed them that if "any work or personal responsibilities" precluded them from returning the survey on the 14th, they could return it to Kirk Fremont's office until October 21. By making the process user-friendly and providing constant encouragement throughout the two-week completion period, the survey conduct team did everything possible to ensure a high response rate and a high level of quality in the data and input provided.

Analysis of the Survey

On October 21, the survey conduct team met to tabulate the total number of survey returns. By waiting a week after the October 14 deadline, Kirk Fremont and his staff collected approximately 50 additional surveys returned after the Friday, October 14, deadline.

Overall Response

Organizationwide, the survey return rate was good. Inclusive of numbers from all four facilities, close to 1,000 employees returned completed surveys—a response rate of approximately 67 percent. The response rates varied slightly from location to location with no significant differences reflecting apathy, discord, or any other negative organizational factor. The survey conduct team, as well as executive management and the board of directors, were quite pleased with the survey response.

As the survey conduct team compiled the results of the survey, they decided that the most expedient way to tabulate the total amount of surveys was to divide the survey returns into packets of 100, creating approximately 10 "packets" of 100 surveys each. Members of the team were then divided into pairs to compile the results. Professor Anderson demonstrated a "scoreboard" method to be used by all team members for easy survey tabulation. Additionally, survey conduct team member Pamela Lauren who worked in the MIS department at Avalon Park Hospital arranged for all team members to utilize personal computers and a simple mathematical software package to tabulate the survey results. Utilizing the methods demonstrated by Professor Anderson and the software innovated by Pamela Lauren, the survey conduct team was able to conduct a complete tabulation of all survey responses by October 28.

Most respondents indicated on the informational sheet which segment of the organization they were a member of and, in many cases, their shift. Approximately 70 percent of the individuals also indicated their department and 60 percent their title. Forty percent of the respondents indicated their name (considered a relatively significant response to this particular question). Most responses of self-identifying individuals were positive.

Comments and Suggestions

The survey conduct team collated the comments and suggestions utilizing a formula of five similar comments/suggestions among each batch of 100 respondents. Additionally, the team noted any personal comments or specific suggestions as per the directions of this text. As a result, five significant issues emerged:

- Lack of adequate intraorganizational communication
- Attitudes of and toward nursing staff
- Lack of cohesive organizationwide identification
- Human resources issues
- General issues

Throughout analysis, the survey conduct team kept Fred Fabian updated via Kirk Fremont.

Lack of Adequate Intraorganizational Communication

Many employees indicated that communication at Avalon Park Hospital and its three "satellite" facilities was not as strong as it could be. For example, many Shileen employees stated that they "did not get the word" on major events at the hospital and upcoming organization projects. This sentiment was supported by responses in section I (relative to the organization). Furthermore, many suggestions and comments written on the final sheet of the booklet addressed the issue of intraorganizational communication from the Avalon Park Hospital to the three outlying facilities.

Attitudes of and toward Nursing Staff

Another major survey outcome touched on issues related to the nursing corps, both from nurses and other employees. Many nurses did respond in full to the survey, and a large percentage provided their name or at least their department. Furthermore, many individuals were identifiable as nurses by virtue of their comments and suggestions. For example, respondents cited particular dynamics of nursing or made statements such as "We RNs feel . . . ," making them easily identifiable as part of the nursing staff.

The major problem as suggested by the survey outcome was that many employees felt as though the nurses were "elitists." Other comments seemed to suggest that many nurses felt they did have a superior position in the organization. Statements by nurses included, "Since we are the hub of the hospital, we should be entitled to more benefits, more pay, and so on. . . ." Other members of the organization made statements such as, "If the nurses don't like working here, if they won't stop complaining, they should go look for work elsewhere" and "If the nurses think they're not being treated correctly or want more pay, they should look at what we do for a living every day." These angry sentiments were echoed with startling resonance in many surveys. In response, the survey conduct team immediately enlisted the participation of Shelly Tyrone, the director of nursing, to review these comments and prepare a potential action plan toward alleviating the problem.

Lack of Cohesive Organizationwide Identification

The third major issue discovered through the survey process was employee lack of identification with the organization's new identity. Many individuals were unaware of the new name Avalon Park Healthcare System or felt this name inadequate because it did not accurately reflect the organization's total scope. Furthermore, a significant number of respondents—about 20 percent overall—made comments along the lines of "Avalon Park is just *one* part of our organization."

The proposed new name was felt by many employees to be proprietary of Avalon Park Hospital—basically "the same wine in a different bottle." Several employees suggested new names. The name suggested most prominently was "The Purple Valley Regional Healthcare System," made by employees from all four facilities.

Human Resources Issues

There seemed to be a particular inclination on the part of survey respondents to assess the human resources department. The survey conduct team noted two main concerns: (1) many individuals felt as though the human resources department did not do enough in terms of education and training; and (2) the issues of compensation levels and benefits administration were called into question by many respondents. Kirk Fremont took particular note of this, and together with Natalie Pine, fellow survey team member and the compensation coordinator, resolved to address these concerns with an action plan.

General Issues

In addition to these four specific issues, the survey conduct team noted several other significant trends. These included:

• The mention of several individuals who had performed outstanding service to the community
• Several ideas relative to customer/patient innovations such as prenatal services to be performed at the clinic and the Shileen facility, in addition to the ongoing program at the Avalon Park facility
• A need for an adult day care center for senior citizens who are dependents of the organization's employees
• An expansion of day care center services for all the organization's members
• The need for additional medical services for teenagers and other young adults with specific medical requirements
• Inclusion of organizational employees in the HMO program

(Many employees of the Avalon Park Hospital were *not* members of the Purple Mountain HMO program. The executive management team registered this as an oversight on their part.)

Action Planning

Once the entire survey analysis was complete, Kirk Fremont and Professor Anderson met with the senior management group to devise action plans. The senior management team looked at the four major critical issues of the survey (each listed independently on a large sheet of paper). For each critical issue, the executive management team arrived at a number of solutions. In addressing the problem of organizationwide identification, for example, the following action plans were discussed:

• Selection of a new name more inclusive of all four facilities
• Distribution of annual reports to members of all four facilities

- Utilization of employee forums in all four facilities to ask for specific ideas on improving identification with the new system
- Utilization of devices such as key chains and coffee cups to increase organizational awareness and identity

As another example, to address the nursing dilemma, Shelly Tyrone felt that a root of the problem was a nurse effectiveness program identifying nursing as "the hub of any hospital." During the conversation, Fred Fabian, as well as other members of the executive management team, made the case that any person who worked at the hospital could be considered the "hub." They cited, for example, a security guard who was instrumental in efficiently and quickly directing someone to the emergency department. Tyrone agreed and decided that perhaps individuals throughout the organization did not know enough about nursing, just as the nursing staff did not know enough about other facets of the organization. With this in mind, one solution to the nursing attitude problem was to increase employees' knowledge of *all* operations by instituting an employee awareness day. It was hoped that this program would help individuals to understand in more depth (and then hopefully respect) the roles their fellow employees play in providing high-quality health care.

The other three issues were discussed in a similar fashion, with five solutions provided for each. Therefore, at the end of this session, the executive management team was armed with 20 potential solutions to the four major dilemmas. Additionally, Fred Fabian took the responsibility to personally execute specific, direct feedback to various organization members. This included passing on compliments to physicians, nurses, and other direct patient care professionals. Fabian did this by sending appreciative letters to each individual and then making personal telephone calls to further thank these individuals for their particular contributions.

Fabian also dealt with several unpleasant situations (employees complaining about a particular manager or a specific unethical practice) that were uncovered by the survey. Both Fabian and Fremont met with the senior managers in charge of the problems to verify the validity of the situations and then come to a resolution.

For example, one extraordinary comment that emerged on a survey centered in the area of responsibility managed by Caitlin Prescott, the chief financial officer. Evidently, one of the accounts receivable clerks felt as though she was not being paid properly for her overtime. She attributed this to her manager "sexually harassing" her on a daily basis, though the problem could have other legal ramifications. Obviously, sexual harassment is an alarming charge and one that any health care management investigation should focus on with the help of legal counsel. Accordingly, Prescott discussed the charge specifically with the accounts receivable manager. In the course of their conversation, Prescott was convinced that the individual who had written the comment was, in fact, being paid correctly for overtime. And since this individual identified herself by name, Prescott decided to discuss the charge with her specifically. When Prescott brought the woman making the allegation into her office for a private conference, the woman denied that she even wrote the comment and stated that "someone else might have done this to get even with me." When Prescott asked whether the woman had any idea who might have done something like that, the woman said that she did not. Prescott reaffirmed the organization's commitment to maintain a fair and equitable workplace and assured the woman that if any other problem ensued relative to sexual harassment or any other lack of workplace fairness that she should bring it directly to Prescott's attention. The woman, quite embarrassed at this point, thanked Prescott for her support and left her office. Although Prescott was somewhat befuddled by the outcome of this case, she felt assured that there was no harassment problem in the workplace. She reported the results of her investigation to Fabian, as did all senior managers, each of whom had at least one allegation to investigate.

To bring the survey process to a close, employee forums were scheduled for the first two weeks of December. Because of the winter holidays, a two-week span was considered an appropriate amount of time to give everyone the opportunity to attend a meeting. During the presentations, Fabian (or another member of the management staff) presented the four major issues identified from the survey and offered their five suggested action plans. The employees were asked to vote on the options for each major issue and/or to provide additional solutions of their own.

The forums proved to be rewarding for the entire organization. In the course of the briefings, attended by approximately 700 members of all four facilities, the following 10 survey outcomes were determined:

1. A preferred new organization name, "The Purple Mountain Regional Healthcare System," was suggested. This name, approved overwhelmingly by employees, was accepted by the board in a February meeting. Accordingly, a new logo was designed that incorporated the new name. Also, all the facilities were renamed to reflect the change. The Avalon Park Hospital became the Purple Mountain Medical Center; the clinic became the Purple Mountain Health Clinic; the Home for the Aging became the Purple Mountain Home for the Aging; and the Shileen Health Facility became the Purple Mountain Health Center. (See figure 6-4.) Changes were made on signage at all facilities and on all stationery, forms, promotional items (coffee cups, for example), and so on.
2. Fremont initiated a major human resources overhaul guided by suggestions derived from both the survey and the subsequent meetings. Changes in human resources administration included the implementation of a new educational program to help all employees become aware of the system's new strategic directions. Also, Fremont established a new employee orientation training program for all levels of the organization.

Figure 6-4. New Purple Mountain Organization

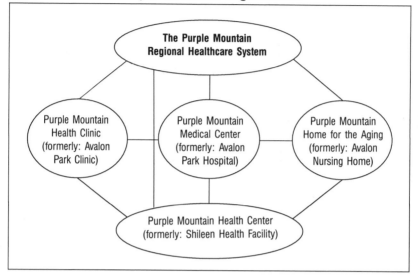

3. Committees composed of both employees and managers were formed to look into the feasibility of extending the existing day care programs and to introduce an adult day care program to be managed by the Home for the Aging. Because the Home for the Aging had a considerable amount of unutilized space and the Purple Mountain HMO Corporation sees the underwriting of an adult care program "in their best interest," this service may become a reality in the near future.

4. A wage survey would be conducted to identify areas of compression not only in compensation differences among the four facilities, but throughout the entire region (a 50-mile radius because that is as far as individuals would go to seek new employment). By June 1st, Fremont would present the comprehensive wage survey to all employees and mandate any wage adjustments organizationwide as appropriate.

5. A pay-for-performance evaluation and compensation system would be implemented in the following year. This progressive human resources program, coupled with the wage survey, would ensure that all individuals are being paid fairly. It would also help ensure that the organization would retain only the best employees.

6. The hospital would implement a new system to garner employee suggestions on a more regular basis. Suggestion boxes would be placed in all four facilities. A "bounty" of $100 would be awarded for any suggestion potentially able to be implemented in the organization. In the eyes of senior management and the employees, this was a stellar example of truly implementing a quality program within a health care facility.

7. Visitor cards would be distributed in all four facilities to every customer/patient utilizing services. Information from these cards will help establish a data base of customer/patient concerns and needs. Establishing such a data base was suggested in the briefing session following the survey. Customer/patients would be asked their opinions on the quality of services and the need for more services and would be offered the opportunity to make suggestions on enhancing the general efficiency and effectiveness of the new Purple Mountain Regional Healthcare System.

8. The human resources staff would look into internal promotions and job transfers at all four facilities. This would help galvanize the organization into a more cohesive, interactive entity, as well as present many more promotional opportunities than currently exist within the organization.

9. The human resources department would present an employee referral recruitment program to help alleviate the pressing need for obtaining more qualified job candidates within nursing and other critical areas.

10. Senior management would have regular monthly meetings with employees to discuss pertinent issues. Though Fred Fabian previously held such meetings, the new process will include inviting the use of a different executive manager each month so that critical issues concerning each organizational segment could be discussed.

Thanks to the survey, the organization now has action plans for the future.

Conclusion

This case study illustrates the attitude survey process undertaken by one fictional health care organization, describing what could and has happened in certain institutions. Obviously, each institution will have its own objectives and concerns when considering and/or conducting an attitude survey. This book addressed those issues both generally and specifically through discussion of the survey system's overview and organizational applications, as well as survey planning and communication. Survey distribution, collection, tabulation, analysis, and action planning were also examined, and the discussion of them was enhanced by the information in the appendixes—a sample survey instrument, survey analysis guides, supplemental survey questions, and a sample organizational action plan.

Appendix A

The Health Care Organizational Survey

Each section of the survey instrument reproduced here and discussed throughout the book contains 10 critical items and is augmented by a section for additional comments and suggestions. The scale on the survey is as follows: SA = strongly agree, A = agree, N = neutral, D = disagree, and SD = strongly disagree. In addition, there is a sample cover letter that can be used in any health care organization's survey booklet. Readers who have questions about the survey instrument are invited to call the author at CHR/ InterVista (telephone: 908/850-0712).

MEMORANDUM

To: All Hospital Managers and Employees
From:
Date:

Subject: Organizational Attitude Survey

With the recent changes and dynamic growth of our organization, it is vital to make certain that we get as many suggestions and insights from our organization members as possible. This is particularly important at this point in the hospital's history, as we face new challenges and an era of change in American health care.

We need your participation in this survey process for several reasons. First, your input and ideas will help us plan major organizational activities for the future. Second, this is a first step in innovating and implementing new human resources and employee relations programs. Finally, taking care of people means taking care of *our* people. With that in mind, we're vitally interested in your suggestions for making our organization a great place to work and grow as a health care professional.

We, at the executive level, absolutely guarantee two things relative to this survey. First, the survey will provide you with complete confidentiality. The results will be collected and reviewed confidentially. Second, we will provide each of you with the opportunity to attend a briefing session regarding the survey results and new action plans based on those results. We will also give all organization members a printed copy of the results.

Please participate fully by completing the form thoughtfully and in its entirety and then returning it. Thank you for helping us to make our organization realize its full potential.

I. THE ORGANIZATION

Take into consideration your view of the entire organization.

1. Considering the changes in the manner in which health care is provided (for example, the shift from inpatient to outpatient care) and growth in our service area, our organization still works to maintain a caring/family atmosphere. SA A N D SD

2. Our organization seems prepared and ready to succeed in meeting the various challenges of the future. SA A N D SD

3. Our organization is one in which ethical action is encouraged and expected from employees and departments. SA A N D SD

4. Our organization's current plans for growth are well conceived, realistic, and reflective of the emerging needs of our community. SA A N D SD

5. Communication efforts are usually clear and timely. SA A N D SD

6. Employees' opinions and input are generally valued, accepted, and acted on appropriately throughout the organization. SA A N D SD

7. Our organization hires new employees who, for the most part, are competent, caring, and committed to quality. SA A N D SD

8. Considering most health care facilities in our geographical area, I would consider our organization a "winner." SA A N D SD

9. In response to the needs of our service area, our organization is responsive and fair in most cases. SA A N D SD

10. Given the change, growth, and other "new dimensions" of our organization and health care in general, I feel that we are in good shape. SA A N D SD

Comments, suggestions, and insights regarding our organization and additional remarks based on the preceding items:

_____

_____

_____

II. THE ORGANIZATION'S MANAGEMENT

Rate the following statements on the basis of your experience with your own immediate supervisor, manager, or director.

1. My manager or supervisor is sensitive to my professional needs and is supportive of my work efforts.   SA A N D SD

2. I am provided with clear direction and goals for achievement most of the time in my position.   SA A N D SD

3. My manager or supervisor understands and appreciates the challenges of my job.   SA A N D SD

4. Crisis, conflict, and differences of opinion are usually handled quickly and effectively in my work area.   SA A N D SD

5. My suggestions and input are truly listened to, not just heard or politely tolerated.   SA A N D SD

6. Quality is generally at the forefront of my manager's or supervisor's plans and is emphasized in every work goal.   SA A N D SD

7. My manager or supervisor uses a leadership style that is motivating and positive most of the time.   SA A N D SD

8. My manager or supervisor is able to implement training for new procedures and work approaches.   SA A N D SD

9. My manager or supervisor makes most critical decisions accurately and in a timely fashion.   SA A N D SD

10. My manager or supervisor encourages cooperation with other departments and helps my efforts to cooperate with other departments.   SA A N D SD

Comments or suggestions for improving managerial action in your area and additional, specific comments based on the preceding items:

_____

_____

_____

III. THE JOB

Take into consideration your current position and daily activities.

1. I have most of the resources I need to do my job in a high-quality manner and at an appropriate quality level.　　SA A N D SD

2. I receive an appropriate amount of training and development relative to my job.　　SA A N D SD

3. I understand how my job fits into the organization's "big picture" and the importance of what I do on a daily basis.　　SA A N D SD

4. The relationship between the people in my department and the medical staff is relatively positive.　　SA A N D SD

5. My job description adequately reflects 60 to 80 percent of my job and its regular ongoing responsibilities.　　SA A N D SD

6. I usually have the opportunity to give input and recommendations regarding my job activity.　　SA A N D SD

7. Quality is vital to my job performance and work output.　　SA A N D SD

8. There are solid opportunities in the organization to grow in my particular area of expertise.　　SA A N D SD

9. My current job provides me with a reasonable degree of professional fulfillment and career satisfaction.　　SA A N D SD

10. Overall, I am motivated and interested in my job, my career, and the contribution I make to the organization.　　SA A N D SD

Comments and suggestions relative to your job and its scope of activities based on the preceding items:

_____

_____

_____

IV. THE WORK ENVIRONMENT/GENERAL ISSUES

Take into consideration your general opinions about your work and your workplace.

1. Our organization is "people-oriented," that is, genuinely concerned about patients and employees.   SA A N D SD

2. Most of the people who work here are dedicated and motivated to provide high-quality health care.   SA A N D SD

3. Most of the people I work with "know their stuff," have a good degree of expertise, and are up-to-date in their field.   SA A N D SD

4. Most of the people I work with are proud of our organization and believe in its goals, objectives, and philosophies.   SA A N D SD

5. Most of my colleagues are relatively motivated and satisfied with the organization and their work roles.   SA A N D SD

6. My pay level is fair considering my job role.   SA A N D SD

7. Mediocre/marginal performance is not tolerated within the organization.   SA A N D SD

8. If a conflict arises on the job between my manager and myself, there are ways available in the organization for a resolution.   SA A N D SD

9. Generally speaking, most work efforts at our organization are pursued in a quality-conscious, cost-effective manner.   SA A N D SD

10. Considering my employment status, the organization provides a satisfactory benefits package.   SA A N D SD

Comments and suggestions relative to your work environment or other general issues:

_____

_____

_____

What additional suggestions, comments, ideas, or specific statements would you like to offer?

_____

_____

_____

V. MANAGEMENT SUPPLEMENT

Take into consideration your role as a manager or supervisor in the organization.

1. Overall, a credible team spirit exists among the management community at our organization.   SA A N D SD

2. Considering everyday dynamics, a relatively positive relationship exists between the management group and the medical staff.   SA A N D SD

3. Management development is a sound part of the organizational system and my professional life here.   SA A N D SD

4. Opportunities exist for needed technical training for both my staff and myself.   SA A N D SD

5. I believe that reasonable measures are being taken to understand employee needs and their key areas of concern.   SA A N D SD

6. Good communication exists between administration and the management team and is consistent, timely, and equally participative.   SA A N D SD

7. The entire organization is progressive and growth-oriented.   SA A N D SD

8. Our organization seems to be well structured and clearly established in the community and, in general, has a "pretty good reputation."   SA A N D SD

9. I feel that the organization provides its employees with a good sense of security and professional stability.   SA A N D SD

10. The organization's future plans, goals, and objectives are publicized throughout the organization in an effective manner.   SA A N D SD

As a member of the organization's management team, what additional insights, comments, or suggestions would you like to add to this survey?

_____

_____

_____

Appendix B

The Survey Analysis Guides

These survey analysis guides can be used by the survey conduct team and reviewing executives to interpret the results of the survey. Guides are provided for every section of the health care organizational survey, except for section V. Section V contains straightforward items that result in varied results and comments. Therefore, the author suggests using your own collective perceptions and knowledge of the organization to provide an accurate and comprehensive analysis of these items.

Although the analysis guides provide specific information, it is strongly suggested that the survey conduct team and reviewing executives temper the utilization of the analysis guides for sections I through IV with their own perceptions and that in all cases they review the survey results with as many employees and managers as possible to draw clear conclusions and construct solid action plans relative to the survey.

Analysis Guide Section I: The Organization

Item 1

Considering the changes in the manner in which health care is provided (for example, the shift from inpatient to outpatient care) and growth in our service area, our organization still works to maintain a caring/family atmosphere.

Item's Intent: To assess general perceptions on the internal work atmosphere of the entire organization.

Response Indicators and Action Plans:

SA Strong agreement from a significant number of respondents (usually 25 percent or more) indicates that the organization has a strong orientation collectively, as well as a solidly positive work atmosphere. No major action is needed except for publication of this result.

A Agreement at 20 to 35 percent indicates that, for the most part, a strong work atmosphere is present within the organization. This includes a sense of belonging and interdependence among all members of the workforce. Again, no major action is needed.

N Neutral responses from a large majority suggest that a satisfactory number of individuals perceive a sound work atmosphere within the organization. Neutral responses can also indicate that a work atmosphere, particularly as typified by an adjective such as *family* or *team* (the optional language for this statement), is not important to the respondent. This issue could be clarified in debriefing meetings subsequent to the survey or pursued through other human resources actions.

D Disagreement with this particular statement can indicate a dissatisfaction with the work atmosphere throughout the organization. A substantial percentage of disagreement (20 percent or more) signals legitimate cause for alarm to the senior executive management team. Action taken in this case includes:
- Specific organizational intervention strategies, such as team building, consulting, and other organizational development programs
- A close, interpersonal audit of the entire organization (particularly any factions that might have responded negatively to this statement)
- An examination of any recent, significant change that has affected the entire organization and reevaluation of the employees' reaction to this change

SD Strong disagreement with this statement can indicate strong negativity throughout the organization and/or specific work groups or departments. It can also indicate that problems with morale are present in several departments. The causes for this strong disagreement should be evident in responses to other parts of the survey.

Item 2

Our organization seems prepared and ready to succeed in meeting the various challenges of the future.

Item's Intent: To provide a clear evaluation, in the opinion of all members of the organization, on the organization's preparedness for current and future health care challenges.

Response Indicators and Action Plans:

SA Strong agreement from a significant percentage (20 percent or more) clearly indicates that most of the strong players in the organization feel that it is ready for all future challenges. This feeling can be reinforced by encouraging the participation of all organization members in strategic and action planning.

A Agreement of 30 percent or more (particularly when combined with a significant percentage of *strongly agree* responses) indicates that employees believe strong organizational preparedness does exist. Again, this feeling can be encouraged through employee participation in strategic and action planning.

N In certain cases, members of the nonexempt workforce may respond in a neutral fashion to this statement because they perceive that the organization's preparedness has little to do with their daily activities. On the other hand, a neutral reaction to this statement may also indicate that certain individuals do not feel they have enough information to respond. Resist the temptation to read too much into this response.

D Disagreement with this statement as represented by a response of 10 percent or more should be investigated in the following manner:
- A second questionnaire could be distributed to various respondents to ask how preparedness could be enhanced.
- Department managers could undertake specific questioning to ask how preparedness could be enhanced.
- Individuals with specific technical expertise could be asked to join a committee or an ongoing quality improvement effort to increase preparedness.
- The organization's suggestion box system could include specific questions on organizational preparedness.
- Customer/patient response could be encouraged through the use of infocards or other feedback mechanisms.

SD Strong disagreement with this statement at 10 percent or more should be investigated. Specific inquiries and investigations can be made to determine whether there is a valid reason for believing the organization is not as prepared as it should be and to establish ways to increase organizational preparedness. Strong disagreement responses to this statement may have specific relevance for organizations where significant change has occurred in the customer/patient environment or where there has been significant internal restructuring.

Item 3

Our organization is one in which ethical action is encouraged and expected from employees and departments.

Item's Intent: To determine whether employees perceive ethical action as a way of life throughout the organization.

Response Indicators and Action Plans:

SA Strong agreement from a significant percentage of respondents (25 percent or more) indicates that ethical action is encouraged throughout the organization and that it is a shared value of all organization members. This response percentage also indicates that executives and managers have done a good job in reinforcing ethical standards throughout the operation and have rewarded those who conduct their jobs professionally and ethically.

A Agreement from a significant percentage (35 percent or more) underscores the *strongly agree* response that ethical action is prized throughout the organization and has value in daily activity. This positive trend should be acted upon in the following manner:
- Continuance of hiring practices that assess the ethical standards and work values of job applicants
- Incorporation of a value-based set of standards for performance evaluation
- The use of ethical action as a theme in all orientation and training and development activities

N Neutral responses of any significant percentage (15 percent or more) usually indicate that ethical action is at a satisfactory level throughout the organization. Most health care employees believe that ethical action is an intrinsic part of their daily responsibilities and so are not predisposed to rating it particularly high. A large neutral rating can be viewed as positive if the remaining majority of responses are in the *agree* and/or *strongly agree* categories.

D Significant disagreement with this statement is measured at 10 percent or more. Because most individuals believe that they *personally* act ethically in providing health care, disagreement with this statement must be investigated by all managers and executives to elicit specific examples of departures from ethical action. This investigation should be done quickly and thoroughly.

SD Strong disagreement at any significant percentage (7 percent or more) indicates that the organization may need to take significant action to discover what actions are perceived as being unethical by a segment of the employee population. The reviewing executives should try to identify among themselves what this negative action might have been and then validate that opinion with employees and other professionals in the organization in employee forums and survey debriefing sessions. Discovering and resolving these issues should also be pursued by human resources specialists and other professionals involved in the survey action.

Item 4

Our organization's current plans for growth are well conceived, realistic, and reflective of the emerging needs of our community.

Item's Intent: To solicit employees' opinions on whether the organization is growing in the right direction as far as its growth plans and future objectives.

Response Indicators and Action Plans:

SA Strong agreement with this statement is 15 percent or more. Because this statement asks not only for the employees' perception of the growth plans but for their participation in determining plans for growth and future development, a high percentage of strong agreement with this statement is unlikely. Only a certain percentage of the organization's members truly participate in the planning and development process.

A In a healthy organization, agreement with this statement is 40 percent or more. The average health care employee needs to understand the organization's growth plans only to feel a sense of security and stability relative to them. In other words, having knowledge of growth plans helps enhance employees' job satisfaction, employment security, and continued service to the community. Agreement with this statement is a realistic expectation for most health care organizations that have done an adequate job of communicating their growth plans and future development objectives.

N Strong health care organizations usually see a neutral response rate to this statement ranging from 15 to 25 percent. Again, most employees have a basic understanding of the organization's growth plans but feel that these plans have no specific relevance to their jobs. Therefore, they truly feel neutral in regard to this statement. Furthermore, some organizations enjoy a steady, progressive growth rate (although this is beginning to become more the exception than the rule in modern American health care) and thus the statement is almost meaningless to certain rank-and-file employees.

D   Disagreement with this statement is considered significant in the range
    of 20 to 30 percent or more. If such a percentage is evidenced in response
    to this statement, several issues may be negatively affecting the organi-
    zation. These issues, along with action plans to eliminate their possible
    negative effects, include:
    • A lack of communication relative to the action plans and future growth
      of the organization indicates a need for management to be more
      specific and complete in its communication with employees about
      growth plans.
    • Illustrations of the growth plans should be presented to the employees,
      possibly including architectural drawings showing plans for a new
      wing, pie charts illustrating patient census increases, or other graphic
      tools. Such illustrations can be presented to employees in forums or
      publications (weekly newsletters, for example).
    • Employee involvement in presenting growth plans to all members of
      the organization should be encouraged. Although it is not essential (and
      in some cases not feasible) to have employees participate in the develop-
      ment of growth plans, it is always possible and valuable to have them
      participate in deciding how these plans will be communicated.
SD Strong disagreement with this statement (around 10 percent) indicates
    direct disagreement with the organization's growth plans. However, em-
    ployees who disagree usually do not completely understand the growth
    plans of the organization or have become aware of the plans only through
    rumor or innuendo. Individuals who strongly disagree with this state-
    ment are those who feel as though the organization is moving in the
    wrong direction. Organization executives should not worry if the num-
    ber of respondents who strongly disagree is 10 percent or less. Often,
    these individuals probably disagree with most of the organization's plans
    and objectives. If more than 10 percent strongly disagree, executive
    management should determine whether the organization's growth plans
    may cause "negative fallout" with a particular segment of the employee
    population.

Item 5

Communication efforts are usually clear and timely.

Item's Intent: To assess basic employee reaction to the quality of communication throughout the organization and to determine whether most individuals
feel as though they get needed information on a timely basis.

Response Indicators and Action Plans:

SA A significant strong agreement percentage for this statement is 10 per-
    cent or more. Because the average American has been bombarded with

an assortment of psychobabble books relative to the communication process, most respondents can think of at least one incident or individual circumstance where communication was not generated efficiently or to their liking. Because interpersonal communication is a highly personal issue, a personal response is usually generated. Therefore, the subjective nature of the response may lead to a lower than average response rate to strong agreement on this statement.

A   Agreement with this statement is 30 percent or more, indicating that most steady, strong contributors in the organization feel communication is a useful tool and valued commodity. In essence, individuals are indicating that most of the time communication is generated in a timely, thoughtful, and efficient manner. Again, given the nature of this statement, it is unrealistic to expect response in the *agree* category to be higher than 30 percent.

N   In many cases, neutral response to this statement is 35 percent or more, even in the best organizations. Because communication is an expected *need* of the health care work relationship, it takes on a "pass/fail" perspective. Accordingly, an organization should be very pleased to receive a "pass" designation on this statement.

D   Disagreement with this statement should be less than 25 percent. If disagreement were more than 25 percent, the following steps might be taken:
   • Establishment of communication awareness programs throughout the organization for all staff members
   • Establishment of communication training programs for all management team members
   • Increased use of organizational communication techniques, such as Friday afternoon forums, newsletters, and employee council meetings
   • Increased communication among the executive committee and staff and all managers and employees
   • Specific action programs targeted at enhancing communication on organizational issues, new projects, and objectives

SD Strong disagreement with this statement is alarming at 10 percent or more. As stated previously, at least 10 percent of the employees will complain about anything, and communication is an obvious issue about which they can express dissatisfaction. If the response in the *strongly disagree* category is more than 10 percent, quickly and effectively implement the strategies indicated in the *disagree* category. If less than 10 percent, simply chalk up the strong disagreement to human behavior.

Item 6

Employees' opinions and input are generally valued, accepted, and acted on appropriately throughout the organization.

Item's Intent: To determine whether employees feel that their input is valued and acted on by organization leadership.

Response Indicators and Action Plans:

SA Strong agreement with this statement (again, because it is related to communication) is rarely more than 5 percent. Some health care executives feel that the phrase "acted on" is what drives this percentage down. Although this could be the case in certain organizations, in general, communication is the central issue here. "Acted on" can simply mean that the employee's suggestion receives some kind of feedback, even if it is a well-considered no. Employees feel that the opportunity to participate and communicate honestly in the work relationship is a necessity. Therefore, the statement takes on the same pass/fail characteristic as item 5.

A A good agreement percentage with this statement (35 percent or more) clearly indicates that employees have the opportunity to participate in the direction of the organization and that their input is respected.

N Neutral response percentage to this statement is the benchmark response. Neutral responses can be positive. However, employees' sense that their opinions are listened to and valued can be further enhanced through additional mechanisms (especially employee–management forums) to garner employee input and suggestions.

D Disagreement with this statement at a rate of 25 percent or more indicates that, for the most part, employees feel disenfranchised from the organization. This response rate is a definite cause for alarm, and to address it the executive management should immediately take the following steps:

- Direct the human resources staff to review any and all existing employee communication mechanisms.
- Direct managers to emphasize employee opportunity to participate in meetings and daily activities.
- Include the CEO and other executive staff members in a variety of efforts to garner employee input.
- Create employee committees in specific areas and enhance ongoing quality improvement efforts that will increase employee communication participation.

SD Strong disagreement with this statement (at a rate of 10 percent or more) indicates that the steps outlined in the disagree category should be taken immediately. Any response of less than 10 percent probably represents small-scale employee dissatisfaction with management's failure to follow a specific suggested action. In this case, management can reevaluate certain employee suggestions to emphasize to employees *why* certain suggested ideas would not be beneficial to the organization.

Item 7

Our organization hires new employees who, for the most part, are competent, caring, and committed to quality.

Item's Intent: To evaluate the quality of newly hired employees, an issue that has obvious value to determining organizational morale, readiness, and effectiveness.

Response Indicators and Action Plans:

SA Strong agreement with this statement is 10 percent or more. Most employees will not rave about new hires, unless there has been a dramatic increase in the quality of new hires over a recent time period. Furthermore, most employees *expect* that the organization will hire individuals who are at least as competent as existing staff. Therefore, it is more likely that respondents will strongly agree with or even be neutral to this statement if they feel that the organization is doing a good job in selecting new employees.

A In many cases, agreement with this statement is 50 to 70 percent. Most employees feel that the organization is good, if not great, if it hires individuals with talent, compassion, and determination to provide high-quality health care. Therefore, agreement with this statement is an endorsement that new hires are at least as competent as the more long-term staff. Additionally, new hires are participating in the survey; therefore, it is only natural that they would rate themselves at least better than satisfactory.

N Neutral response to this statement between 10 to 30 percent is satisfactory. In certain cases, some individuals may be neutral because their departments have not hired anyone new for a significant period of time.

D If there is wide-scale disagreement with this statement (20 percent or more), the organization should immediately take the following steps:
- Conduct an audit of existing human resources and employee selection processes to determine lapses in quality or lack of expertise on the part of recruitment specialists and others involved in the selection process.
- Implement a structured selection process to ensure quality.
- Consult resources to increase knowledge in this area.
- Determine whether recruitment sources (such as agencies) are doing their job adequately.
- Compare performance evaluation data and hiring data to determine whether new hires are truly qualified.
- Rotate interview strategies, panel strategies, and other recruitment strategies.

SD Strong disagreement (10 percent or more) mandates an immediate implementation of the steps discussed in the *disagree* category. An additional strategy is to utilize employee referrals. The success of this strategy depends on the use of a good job-posting system; an effective human resources department; and development of clear standards for employee recruitment, selection, and orientation.

Item 8

Considering most health care facilities in our geographical area, I would consider our organization a "winner."

Item's Intent: To determine the employees' perception of the organization's position with respect to the surrounding environment and customer/patient community.

Response Indicators and Action Plans:

SA Strong agreement with this statement is 25 percent or more. Most employees, even if dissatisfied with other aspects of the organization, still feel as though the organization is a winner. Put simply, if individuals do not strongly believe that their organization is trying to be successful and progressive, they would probably be seeking employment elsewhere. This feeling is particularly strong for managers and professionals, because, despite geographical region or need for relocation, there are usually more opportunities for them.

A In most solid health care organizations, agreement with this statement at a rate of 40 percent or more is a very healthy sign. In this case, a suitable action plan is to identify the reasons why most employees feel that their perception of the organization is positive and to use those building blocks in all future efforts.

N Neutral response of 10 percent or more is common for two basic reasons. First, most individuals feel that the organization simply rates "satisfactory" in this regard. Employee satisfaction can be enhanced, however, through a variety of organizational programs, as well as through increasing the flow of information about organizational activities, upcoming events, and long-range objectives. The second reason for this lower percentage is the higher percentages in the *strongly agree* and *agree* categories. Often, the nonplayers in the organization select neutral as part of ongoing contentious behavior. However, a large neutral response (usually 20 percent or more) will be coupled with stronger percentages in the *disagree* and *strongly disagree* categories. If this is the case, follow the action plans prescribed in the *disagree* category.

D Disagreement with this statement at 15 percent is cause for alarm. Put simply, most individuals who disagree with this statement are probably focusing on a major negative issue or issues. It is important for management to use debriefing sessions that encourage open discussion regarding these issues and whether they can be addressed or must be accepted as a "fact of life" in the organization. For example, if the employees feel that a significant recent change in a customer relations program will give the hospital a bad name, this concern should be addressed. As another example, if a hospital is located in a small industrial city whose population has decreased considerably in recent years, many individuals may feel the perception of the hospital is suffering because of a decrease in business. This would fall into the "fact of life" category.

SD Strong disagreement with this statement higher than 10 percent must be addressed immediately. Strong disagreement responses usually appear in organizations that have recently undergone significant change (such as a merger or acquisition). Some individuals feel as though the recent change is a mistake that will hamper the organization's future. Although these feelings need to be addressed, they must be assessed along with the other responses in that particular survey.

Item 9

In response to the needs of our service area, our organization is responsive and fair in most cases.

Item's Intent: To assess the employees' perception of organizational responsiveness to the service area and the quality of care provided to that service area.

Response Indicators and Action Plans:

SA Strong agreement with this statement (10 percent or more) is positive, indicating that most individuals feel the organization is doing an adequate job in this regard. However, unless the organization has a very specific agenda, such as a specialty area or specific customer–patient base, it is difficult for employees to strongly agree with the premise that the organization provides stellar service all of the time. Most health care organizations work in communities and service areas that have constantly changing needs. Additionally, under the present conditions in health care, employees have expectations and demands that are almost impossible to determine, let alone satisfy completely on a daily basis. With this particular statement, the response rate in the *agree* category more accurately represents the employees' perspective.

A Agreement with this statement of 50 percent or more indicates that the organization is responsive to the needs of its customer/patients and is basically achieving its mission. This positive response should be highlighted in postsurvey reports, incorporated into all organizational objectives and training, and emphasized in all briefing meetings. Furthermore, the reasons why this prevailing positive feeling exists should be explored in the debriefing sessions and survey presentations.

N Neutral responses to this statement should be less than 15 percent. Any more than that is not satisfactory because all employees should have a strong sense of whether the needs of the customer community are being met. For example, most individuals who work in a typical community hospital are also citizens of the service community. Therefore, they have clear perspective and definite opinions on whether the needs of the community are being met. Anyone who is neutral in response to this statement may be saying that they simply do not have enough information to make a determination. Such individuals include those who work at the hospital but are not residents of the community, and/or who have very limited or no direct contact with patients.

D   Any disagreement with this statement greater than 7 percent must be investigated immediately. The key questions in the investigation are:
   • Why do you think the organization is not responsive?
   • Do you think it is an internal issue that causes the organization to be nonresponsive?
   • Would you consider the organization to be irresponsible relative to the service area? Why?
   • What would you do if you were in control of the hospital to make it more responsive?
   • What do we need to do in order to make the organization more responsive to the needs of our customer/patients?

   These questions should be posed to any and all organization members who might provide credible, realistic input. Once again, remember that significant recent change in the institution might have skewed individual perceptions in this regard. For example, many individuals may feel that the organization has done a disservice to the community because, due to financial constraints, it had to close a wing of the hospital. Again, however, concern about these issues must be addressed in the interest of ensuring good overall responsiveness to the service community.

SD Strong disagreement with this statement (greater than 5 percent) is considered in concert with the responses in the *disagree* category. Looking at these two categories together gives a strong indication of prevailing negative sentiment. *Strongly disagree* responses are investigated with the same techniques advised in the *disagree* category.

Item 10

Given the change, growth, and other "new dimensions" of our organization and health care in general, I feel that we are in good shape.

Item's Intent: To assess employees' perception of the overall general position of the hospital relative to uncontrollable, external conditions.

Response Indicators and Action Plans:

SA Strong agreement with this statement at 10 percent or more is a positive indicator. Because the statement is broad in nature, the organization should not expect a large response percentage in the *strongly agree* category. Any strong agreement less than 10 percent is taken into consideration with the responses in the other categories.

A Agreement with this statement of 40 percent or more is excellent, indicating that most employees believe that the organization is taking the proper steps to avoid being caught by surprise by any negative environmental force (such as local economic downturns or regional industrial flights or downsizing). These individuals are also indicating they trust the organization to provide high-quality health care.

N Neutral responses may reflect either neutral or satisfactory sentiments in regards to this statement. The neutral response percentage may also act as a swing vote. For example, a 10 percent response rate in the *neutral* category can augment a majority of *agree* and *strongly agree* responses or, conversely, a majority of *disagree* or *strongly disagree* responses. In either case, all category responses must be looked at before making a final determination of what the neutral responses represent.

D Disagreement with this statement exceeding 20 percent is a bad sign. Reasons for disagreement may be related to any one of the preceding nine items in this section—the Organization. Action plans should be drawn, as appropriate, from analysis guides in this as well as other sections of the survey. The organization must determine why individuals perceive the general position of the organization as weak. Rooted in the *why* should be the potential solutions for increasing the employees' perceptions positively in regard to this statement.

SD Strong disagreement with this statement at more than 10 percent reinforces the negative perceptions presented in the *neutral* and/or *disagree* categories. The action plan utilized to counteract the negativity is the same one suggested in the *disagree* category. In cases where the *strongly disagree* response is very significant (such as 20 percent), it is likely that responses to all items in this section were also strongly disagreed with, indicating a need for significant organizational change and increased efforts in the areas of employee relations, organizational development, and human resource management.

Analysis Guide Section II:
The Organization's Management

Item 1

My manager or supervisor is sensitive to my professional needs and is supportive of my work efforts.

Item's Intent: To assess respondents' perception relative to the amount of sensitivity and support demonstrated by their manager or supervisor on a daily basis.

Response Indicators and Action Plans:

SA Strong agreement with this statement (20 to 30 percent) indicates that management training has been effective in teaching managers to be communicative with and supportive of employees. It also indicates that there is a certain degree of allegiance from employees to their managers and to the organization as a whole.

A Agreement from a significant majority (usually between 35 to 45 percent) indicates that the management group as a whole is well trained, sensitive to the needs of the employees, and capable of working with employees toward progressive objectives. It also indicates that the organization's training and management development programs are successful and that most employees (certainly the strong players and steady players) feel that their managers are genuinely interested in their well-being and professional development.

N Neutral responses to this statement may appear for various reasons. A neutral response can mean that the employee is not particularly motivated by his or her manager. It can also mean that the employee perceives his or her work role as autonomous to a certain degree; that is, the employee does not *need* a lot of management support or sensitivity in order to accomplish daily goals. Additionally, a neutral response can indicate that the employee is simply not the type of person that wants a lot from his or her manager. Rather, he or she merely wants enough resources and independence to complete his or her goals.

On the other hand, some individuals select the *neutral* category because they have not heretofore considered the issue of interpersonal dynamics relative to their manager. Or, in certain cases, a neutral response to this statement means an uneven perception of managerial support and sensitivity. That is, the manager might have been sensitive and supportive in some cases, but not in others.

D Disagreement of 20 percent or more with this statement indicates negative sentiment toward the entire management team. A percentage this large in the *disagree* category is usually augmented by a response rate of 15 percent or more in the *strongly disagree* category (further underscoring that many employees feel that their managers are not sensitive or supportive of their efforts). For example, if the response rate in the *disagree* category is 20 percent, but the response rate in the *strongly disagree* category is less than 10 percent, then there is a likelihood that most nonplayers have responded negatively to the statement. However, if the *strongly disagree* percentage is the same or higher than the *disagree* percentage, that indicates that some steady players also perceive a problem with managerial support and sensitivity. In this case, new efforts in management training and development focused on interpersonal relations with employees should be instituted or redirected.

SD In the case of strong disagreement with this statement (15 percent or more), the survey analysis team should review possible reasons for this negativity. A certain amount of significant change that took place in the organization may have been perceived as negative or managers may have had to deal with circumstances and change largely out of their control. Another reason could be that employees perceive management as being insensitive and nonsupportive due to labor relations issues or other organizational dynamics. The survey conduct team reviews the recent history of the organization and determines whether the responses in the *strongly disagree* category are indicative of current events or those in the recent past. If there are no significant issues in the recent past or at present that might skew response to this statement, then the survey conduct team has to assume that a problem exists in management training and overall manager sensitivity to employees. In this case, certain organizational training and development efforts must be implemented immediately.

Item 2

I am provided with clear direction and goals for achievement most of the time in my position.

Item's Intent: To assess the employees' perception of their managers' provision of clear and ongoing standards and objectives. The definition of ongoing standards and objectives by managers is critical to the employees' success as well as the maintenance of the work groups' motivation and morale.

Response Indicators and Action Plans:

SA Strong agreement with this statement is usually never more than 10 to 15 percent because the large amount of change that takes place within a typical health care organization makes it difficult for a manager to always provide clear direction and goals to the employee. Therefore, unless the organization has a high degree of stability and security, strong agreement with this statement is usually low—often the lowest of the 10 statements in this section.

A   In most progressive health care organizations, agreement with this statement is usually 30 to 45 percent. In this case, most employees feel that their managers provide specific objectives on a daily basis, as well as more general departmental and organizational goals.

N   Even in the best health care organizations, neutral response to this statement ranges from 10 to 30 percent. Again, the omnipresence of change has a great deal to do with how the employees respond. For example, some employees remember a recent work experience in which they failed to receive clear direction or goals from their manager. Additionally, goals in health care organizations often change quickly (in response to customer/ patient demands, for example). Therefore, it is difficult for employees in some organizations to respond better than neutral to this statement.

D   Disagreement with this statement at 15 percent or more usually indicates that managers and supervisors need to display more effort in providing work goals and direction for employees.

SD Strong disagreement with this statement (10 percent or more) indicates problems within the organization. Although many nonplayers strongly disagree with many of the positively positioned statements in the survey, if an organization receives this percentage of strong disagreement, it should take the following actions:

- Reinforce management training (including sessions on how to present goals and document performance).
- Ask employees to give specific examples of when they were not provided clear work direction on an individual basis.
- Allow managers to offer their own suggestions on how work goals might be presented more thoughtfully. (This can be accomplished easily in the action plans and postsurvey feedback meetings.)

Item 3

My manager or supervisor understands and appreciates the challenge of my job.

Item's Intent: To determine how much employees believe their manager understands the employees' jobs and work roles.

Response Indicators and Action Plans:

SA In most progressive health care organizations, strong agreement with this statement is usually 15 percent or more because most managers have held positions similar to the employees' prior to promotion into management. Therefore, managers understand the employees' daily responsibilities and work roles.

A In most solid health care organizations, agreement with this statement is 35 percent or more indicating that most employees feel their manager at least understands what they do on a daily basis (both technical and nontechnical) and that their manager shows a certain amount of ongoing empathy and understanding.

N Neutral response to this statement is usually less than 20 percent. The major reason an individual responds neutrally to this statement is that he or she identifies one particular aspect of his or her job or a particular event that in his or her perception the manager did not understand or fully recognize. For further clarification, it is hoped that the employee who responds neutrally to this statement writes specific comments in the comments and suggestion section of the survey instrument.

D Disagreement with this statement greater than 20 percent indicates a negative situation in the health care organization. Individuals who disagree with this particular statement believe that the manager has no basic understanding of the employees' job. It is vital that managers have a clear understanding of what their employees do on a given day, not only for proper performance evaluation and other managerial responsibilities, but also to ensure that the employees are being fully utilized. If disagreement with this statement is significant, managers and supervisors should reorient themselves about their employees' responsibilities and daily activities.

SD Strong disagreement with this statement (10 percent or more) indicates that the actions suggested in the *disagree* category should be taken immediately. Furthermore, encourage managers to spend a day or two with the particular employee, asking questions relative to daily conduct of his or her duties and the needs of the employee to accomplish his or her job at an optimum level.

Item 4

Crisis, conflict, and differences of opinion are usually handled quickly and effectively in my work area.

Item's Intent: To assess the employees' perception relative to management's handling of crisis and conflict in a positive manner.

Response Indicators and Action Plans:

SA Strong agreement with this statement is usually never more than 15 to 20 percent because crises occur so frequently within a health care organization that it is impossible to achieve a perfect rating in every crisis situation. If a management team receives a response in the *strongly agree* category of 20 to 30 percent (or more), the team should not be in health care, but in international diplomacy.

A   Agreement with this statement in the range of 30 to 40 percent is outstanding, indicating that, for the most part, differences are resolved quickly and crisis situations handled adroitly. If this is the case, all of the mechanisms used to train the management team are obviously paying dividends to the organization. Crisis management is one of the most important responsibilities of a modern health care manager, and the resolution of conflict is the second (after the delivery of high-quality health care).

N   Neutral response to this statement is usually 20 percent or more. An employee remembers at least one conflict or crisis that was not resolved to his or her satisfaction. Therefore, he or she gives this statement neither a positive nor a negative rating. The remembered situation is offset by other instances when the manager reacted appropriately and positively.

D   Any disagreement with this statement of 15 percent or more is addressed immediately by training managers in crisis management. In addition, many health care organizations provide training and development courses in conflict resolution and change management. This training should be done in *all* health care organizations, not just in those that register significant disagreement with this statement.

SD In many organizations, strong disagreement with this statement is no more than 10 percent. For the most part, employees understand that the emphasis of this statement is on the *effort* of the manager in resolving crisis and dealing with change. Unless employees feel that managers are truly not interested in resolving crisis effectively, they will not select this category. However, if the response rate in the *strongly disagree* category is more than 10 percent, the organization should immediately enact the suggestions offered in the *disagree* category.

Item 5

My suggestions and input are truly listened to, not just heard or politely tolerated.

Item's Intent: To assess employees' reactions to the amount of input they are allowed to provide their managers, and their evaluation of the managers' reactions to that input.

Response Indicators and Action Plans:

SA Strong agreement with this statement at 15 percent or more is excellent. Most organizations pride themselves on allowing employees the opportunity to provide input on certain issues. One of the values of the recent quality management training undertaken in many health care organizations is the encouragement of all employees to provide input when appropriate.

A   Agreement with this statement is as high as 40 to 50 percent in good organizations, indicating that most employees feel they are part of a team dedicated toward providing high-quality health care and that managers are truly interested in employee input regarding this process. Notice that the statement does not discuss whether employee input is acted on, but rather whether it is allowed, facilitated, and considered (a reasonable expectation of any health care professional).

N   Neutral responses to this statement may indicate satisfaction as opposed to ambivalence or neutrality. A response rate in the *neutral* category exceeding 25 percent should be assessed as satisfactory. However, a small percentage of individuals who select the neutral response to this statement are simply not interested in providing suggestions or opinions to their managers and therefore have no interest or basis from which to evaluate this statement.

D   Disagreement with this statement at 15 percent or more indicates that the communication strategies utilized by the management team should be reassessed, especially if the percentage in the *strongly disagree* category is also high.

SD Strong disagreement with this statement is considered critically negative if greater than 10 percent. This situation usually occurs at organizations in which employees have poor morale and there is the possibility of unionization or other potentially stressful developments. In this case, organizational leadership should take greater interest in the employees' suggestions and further encourage them to provide input. Additionally, quality improvement programs and other communication-based training should be implemented immediately. Not encouraging employee feedback and suggestions may cause not only employee resentment, but missed improvement opportunities for the organization.

Item 6

Quality is generally at the forefront of my manager's or supervisor's plans and is emphasized in every work goal.

Item's Intent: To determine employees' perception of quality throughout the organization generally and in their work group specifically, as encouraged by managers and supervisors.

Response Indicators and Action Plans:

SA Strong agreement with this statement is usually 15 percent or more. Because most employees are well aware of the push for quality initiatives in health care organizations, they need no precise definition of quality or its implications in the health care forum. Therefore, employees are usually willing to make a clear determination of their supervisors' commitment to quality. Additionally, employees are well qualified in the idea of quality objectives and the use of quality terminology, so that they are able to recognize whether their manager is truly committed to quality in performing his or her daily responsibilities.

A Agreement with this statement may exceed 45 percent in good health care organizations. Most employees basically agree with this statement because they feel their managers are personally committed to quality and that commitment is encouraged by the organization. In turn, the managers present quality as a major strategic goal in daily work plans. Because most health care professionals recognize that quality in health care often determines life or death, most health care employees have an innate dedication to quality and seek to have that commitment to quality supported by their managers' actions.

N Neutral response to this statement of 20 percent or more is usually a negative sign, indicating that some employees do not feel that quality is an important issue. It may also indicate that employees know of certain situations where quality was not a major objective, at least in their perception or opinion. Again, most employees will elaborate on specific situations in the comments and suggestions section at the bottom of the page. However, if the neutral percentage rate is 20 percent or more organizationwide, it may be useful to investigate the effects of quality training in the organization as well as to conduct an audit of the implementation of quality standards.

D Disagreement with this statement is usually less than 20 percent. In fact, in most stellar health care organizations, disagreement is less than 10 percent. If there are quality issues in the health care organization, they have probably already been brought to the attention of executive management. No ethical health care professional wants to work in an organization where quality is of secondary importance. Therefore, any disagreement with this statement greater than 20 percent raises a red flag to the organization's executive management.

SD In many health care organizations, this statement receives a strong disagreement response rate of 5 percent or less. In fact, in several attitude surveys the author has conducted in organizations of more than 1,000 employees, no respondent selected the *strongly disagree* category. Because strong disagreement with this statement is an indictment of the organization and its mission, the responses to this statement are critical. Managers are the main implementers of quality standards throughout the organization. Therefore, any strong disagreement with this statement must be closely investigated and resolved as quickly as possible. Otherwise, the organization's provision of health care can be jeopardized.

Item 7

My manager or supervisor uses a leadership style that is motivating and positive most of the time.

Item's Intent: To assess employees' reactions to their managers' leadership style. Although this response is usually a subjective reaction, it is often an objective assessment of the effectiveness of the manager's style as perceived by the employee.

Response Indicators and Action Plans:

SA Because employees have their own opinions about what type of management style they prefer, strong agreement with this statement is usually no more than 20 percent. Therefore, it is impossible to expect consensus on the value of a particular management style or philosophy. However, if 15 percent or more of the respondents strongly agree that their manager's leadership style is effective, then the organization is probably hiring and retaining managers who inspire confidence, trust, and motivation.

A Agreement with this statement is usually at least 25 percent in good organizations because most individuals recognize that their managers are utilizing a style that, even if not to the employees' particular liking or taste, is honest and direct.

N Even in the best health care organization, neutral response to this statement is between 20 and 25 percent because a certain number of individuals (in fact, a quarter of the organization) do not view leadership as an issue. The employees simply look to their managers for direction, for fair assessment of their work, and for resources to obtain their desired work goals. Beyond these requirements, they have no particular opinions or expectations of their managers.

D Disagreement with this statement at 15 percent or more indicates a serious problem — that the leadership style utilized by a number of supervisors and managers is demotivating some employees. The response percentage in the *disagree* category is considered in tandem with the *strongly disagree* percentage. A response rate of 20 percent or more in the *disagree* category along with a response rate of 15 percent or more in the *strongly disagree* category mandate that the actions outlined in the *strongly disagree* category should be followed immediately.

SD If strong disagreement is 15 percent or more (and especially if the response rate in the *disagree* category is over 20 percent) the following actions should be taken:
  • Conduct an organizationwide analysis of the leadership styles utilized by managers and supervisors.
  • Conduct a specific survey relative to leadership style and managerial approach.

- Conduct employee forums to determine the specific dynamics and circumstances causing negative perception of the leadership style utilized by the majority of the managers.
- Prepare a list of the words used by managers to describe negative behavior that the employees react to negatively.
- Incorporate suggestions provided by managers, employees, and other parties relative to how the leadership style can be made more positive.
- Adopt a hiring system that utilizes interview and promotional processes that help identify and select managers and supervisors who will embrace a more motivating and uplifting leadership style (provided that the problem is the managers, not the employees).

Item 8

My manager or supervisor is able to implement training for new procedures and work approaches.

Item's Intent: To determine employees' assessment of their managers or supervisors in educating them regarding specific dimensions of their jobs as well as organizational innovations.

Response Indicators and Action Plans:

SA Strong agreement with this statement is significant at 10 percent or more. However, because an emphasized challenge of health care managers and supervisors in the 1990s is to act as mentors and educators, the percentage in the *strongly agree* category will be higher in most progressive health care organizations (perhaps as high as 20 percent). It is imperative that all supervisors and managers understand their mandate from the organization to act as educators within the work process.

A   Agreement with this statement (at least 30 percent in most progressive health care organizations) signifies that most managers and supervisors have undertaken and been effective in training and educating their employees. The organization should mandate this responsibility to managers and provide them resources to help them carry it out.

N   Neutral response to this statement is usually 25 to 30 percent. There are three main reasons why an individual is neutral to this statement. First, some individuals may never have observed their managers presenting training or developmental activities to the work group. If the education department and other training resources are the sole trainers and developers of employees, the organization runs the risk that these individuals may burn out or be stretched too thin. Therefore, managers should also be responsible for training and developing employees.

Second, in many organizations, managers do not use a participative style in training and developing employees. Many employees are experts at performing certain tasks and thus should be encouraged to take an active role in training and developing other employees' skills. A neutral response to this statement may indicate that the employees have not been utilized fully in this process.

Finally, a neutral response may indicate that some employees are indifferent to their managers' approach to training and development. In this case, there is little that the organization can or should do because certain steady players and nonplayers just are not interested in training and development.

D In most progressive health care organizations, disagreement with this statement is no more than 10 to 15 percent because most individuals recognize that the managers are doing the best job they can in educating and training or at least in facilitating proper employee education and development. If there is a significant amount of response to this statement in the *disagree* or *strongly disagree* category, the following three steps should be taken:

- Institute educational and training programs to help managers become better training facilitators.
- Take specific steps to provide the support and necessary resources for managers as well as increase their training and development activities.
- Include management interaction sessions in in-service programs so that a cooperative approach is taken toward training and development.

SD In most progressive health care organizations, strong disagreement with this statement does not usually exceed 5 percent. Often, strong disagreement greater than 5 percent is simply attributed to the fact that many employees do not need a tremendous amount of training. Sometimes, a manager only needs to guide an employee, not to constantly train and develop him or her. The manager does have an ongoing responsibility, however, to train and develop individuals as new organizational objectives are set and as essential characteristics of a job change. It is the executive leadership's task to ensure that managers understand and fulfill these responsibilities.

Item 9

My manager or supervisor makes most critical decisions accurately and in a timely fashion.

Item's Intent: To assess employees' perception of their managers' ability to make decisions efficiently and effectively on a regular basis.

Response Indicators and Action Plans:

SA Strong agreement with this statement is usually between 15 to 25 percent in stellar health care organizations and 10 to 20 percent in sound health care organizations. Managers are responsible for making a variety of intricate, important decisions throughout the course of the year, and these decisions obviously affect the work life of the employees. Therefore, it is unrealistic to expect a high level of strong agreement with this statement because the manager makes some decisions that not all employees completely agree with or believe are correct.

A Agreement responses with this statement are more representative of employee sentiment. In sound and stellar organizations, agreement is between 35 to 50 percent, indicating that, for the most part, the employees feel they can trust their managers to make the *best* decision given particular circumstances. Accordingly, a response rate of 25 percent or more in the *agree* category indicates that the organization has done a good job encouraging managers to make valuable and appropriate decisions.

N Neutral responses to this statement are difficult to interpret given the complex nature of this statement. A response rate of 20 percent in the *neutral* category usually indicates that the respondent agrees that his or her manager makes decisions that are not harmful to the organization. Do not read too much into neutral responses given to this statement because employee sentiment is more clearly illustrated by the percentages in the *agree* or *disagree* categories.

D Disagreement with this statement is 10 to 15 percent in most good organizations. Again, as with most of the items relative to the organization's management, responses in the *disagree* category must be considered in tandem with responses in the *strongly disagree* category. That is, if the response in the *strongly disagree* category is 10 percent or more, there may be a problem relative to how decisions are made throughout the organization. If there is a significant disagreement or strong disagreement, the organization should ask itself the following questions:
- Has the organization recently made a significant decision that had a negative effect on the employees?
- Has the organization leadership forced managers to make unpopular decisions due to financial hardship or other organizational dynamics?
- Has the organization undertaken several strategies that have not been popular with the employees but were necessary for survival?

   If the answer to any or all of these questions is yes, the percentages of response in the *disagree* and *strongly disagree* categories may be higher.

SD Strong disagreement with this statement is closely interconnected with the *disagree* category. That is, responses in the *strongly disagree* category simply indicate a stronger reaction to the same dynamics discussed in the *disagree* category.

Item 10

My manager or supervisor encourages cooperation with other departments and helps my efforts to cooperate with other departments.

Item's Intent: To assess the employees' perception relative to the amount of cooperation encouraged by their departmental supervisor in working with other departments and fellow professionals.

Response Indicators and Action Plans:

SA Strong agreement with this statement is usually 30 percent or more. Cooperation is extremely important in health care organizations. Because "doing less with more" is a way of life in every health care organization in the United States and Canada, managers must constantly encourage individuals to cooperate with other individuals and departments to achieve common goals.

A Agreement with this statement is usually 40 percent or more in most sound health care organizations. Because organizations are doing more with less in terms of assigned human resources, employees interact with fellow professionals and other departments on a daily basis. Accordingly, any managers who try to prohibit or do not facilitate interaction are quickly identified by employees.

N Neutral response to this statement usually indicates "does not apply to me" rather than "neutral" by definition. For example, a lab technician has less interaction with other departments than does a human resources professional. Accordingly, this statement is not as meaningful for the lab technician as it is for the human resources specialist.

D Disagreement with this statement of more than 15 percent is a negative result, indicating managers are placing barriers that prohibit employees from working with other departments as effectively as possible. It is the survey analysis team's responsibility to determine which managers are causing these problems and then contact the human resources department, which will determine (with the support of organizational leadership) how to correct this behavior. These efforts can be accomplished in follow-up sessions, or by incorporating specific confidential suggestions made in the survey itself.

SD Strong disagreement with this statement greater than 5 percent indicates a problem. Individuals will strongly disagree with this statement only if they believe a major problem exists in their department. As mentioned in the *disagree* category, skillful utilization of the human resources department and other resources should be enacted to determine specifically where the problem exists. There are usually remarks written in the comments and suggestions section that expand on responses to this statement.

The written comments and suggestions may be related to a specific department. Therefore, these issues must be handled in a highly confidential, nonthreatening manner, shared with the specific manager or supervisor by his or her manager or an executive. Executive management should take into consideration the fact that the employees may simply be "out for the manager." There should be a preponderance of comments—perhaps five similar comments from five different respondents—before identifying any trend. This is particularly true of manager–employee relations. Subconscious and secondary motives may be the reason for some of these comments, and those circumstances should be considered prior to presenting feedback or developing an action plan relative to these outcomes.

Analysis Guide Section III: The Job

Item 1

I have most of the resources I need to do my job in a high-quality manner and at an appropriate quality level.

Item's Intent: To assess employees' perception relative to the amount and suitability of resources available to perform their job in a satisfactory or superior manner.

Response Indicators and Action Plans:

SA　Strong agreement with this statement is never greater than 10 percent because the nature of the statement is such that it basically elicits a "satisfactory" or an "unsatisfactory" response. Therefore, the greater percentage of responses are in the *agree* or *disagree* category. Strong agreement only registers in cases where the responding employee has recently been given an extraordinary resource (such as new state-of-the-art technology) to complete his or her job.

A　Agreement with this statement is 60 percent or more in solid health care organizations. Agreement simply reflects that the responding employees feel that they have all the resources *needed* to perform their job functions satisfactorily on a daily basis.

N　Neutral response of 15 percent or less can be considered normal because it is interpreted in two ways. First, many employees *want* more resources than they currently have. Many health care employees are well aware of new and improved methods and equipment for the provision of health care and often point to these methods and technologies on the survey. An employee who feels that there is a different technology or a better way of doing his or her job, but, due to financial or other constraints, has not been afforded these options by the organization, may respond neutrally to this statement.

　　　　Second, many employees select the *neutral* category in response to this statement because they feel satisfied with their job roles and do not have any desire to learn new methods or utilize new equipment.

D　Disagreement with this statement at 15 percent or more may indicate a negative organizational dynamic at work. In this case, the organization should take a serious look at the amount of resources available for individuals and/or specific departments. However, many individuals who disagree with this statement are doing so simply to remain consistent; that is, they are simply disagreeing because they have an axe to grind with the organization as reflected by negative response in the survey overall. As nonplayers, they might not be using the resources that are available.

SD Strong disagreement with this statement at a rate of 5 percent or more indicates a strong distrust of the organization. Strong disagreement greater than 5 percent (and, more critically, greater than 10 percent) with this statement is usually centered in one particular department. For example, all members of the physical therapy department may strongly disagree with this statement. These responses, reviewed with the physical therapy manager, reflect the occurrence of an ongoing discussion relative to the lack of a new equipment or the inability of the organization (as perceived by the members of the department) to provide certain resources that might enable the physical therapists to do their jobs more effectively. Strong results such as this, whether validations or revelations, should be examined closely by the survey conduct team and routed immediately to the appropriate manager.

Item 2

I receive an appropriate amount of training and development relative to my job.

Item's Intent: To assess employees' perception of management support provided as demonstrated by specific job training and professional development opportunities in the individuals' area of technical expertise.

Response Indicators and Action Plans:

SA Strong agreement with this statement greater than 10 percent is extraordinary and usually given by individuals who have received an inordinate amount of specific technical training. However, in many organizations where progressive training development is consistently part of organizational conduct, a percentage greater than 15 is obtainable in the *strongly agree* category. It is important to obtain positive responses to this statement because they indicate that employees feel a certain amount of allegiance to the organization, have a sense of ongoing fulfillment in their jobs, and believe that the organization truly cares about their development as health care professionals.

A Agreement with this statement from a large majority of respondents (more than 60 percent) indicates that the organization has done a good job in upgrading the skills and expertise of organization members. This statement, like many in section 3, receive either a yes or no response. That is, individuals are either satisfied or not with the amount of training and development they receive relative to their jobs. Therefore, percentages in the *agree* or *disagree* categories are the key indicators here.

N Neutral response to this statement of 15 percent or less is considered acceptable by an organization for several reasons. Many jobs in a health care organization do not require tremendous technical or professional training (such as environmental services, security, or volunteer services). Once these employees receive basic on-the-job orientation and complete the first year of employment, they feel they are fully qualified and do not desire or need more training. Additionally, many individuals feel fully competent in performing their jobs and have received performance evaluations attesting to that fact. Therefore, they are neutral relative to the issue of training and development.

Another reason for a neutral response to this statement is an employee's lack of awareness relative to suitable training and development programs. It is the manager's *and* the employee's responsibility to create a training and development plan to further enhance the employee's skills. An action plan to respond to a response rate in the *neutral* category greater than 15 percent is for the organization to encourage managers and supervisors at every level to discuss training and development needs with their employees.

D   Disagreement with this statement greater than 10 percent indicates that some members of the organization do not feel they are receiving the proper training and development. A large rate of disagreement (in this case, 20 percent or more) is cause for alarm and should alert the education department and other applicable entities to double their efforts toward increasing employee training and development. Any response of 10 percent or less in the *disagree* category is interpreted to be chronic complaining as verified by examining individual surveys and finding a pattern of disagreement with all positive statements. Many employees who disagree with this statement feel that it is solely the responsibility of the organization and its managers to provide training and development. They simply use this statement as another example of why the organization "doesn't care about me."

SD Strong disagreement with this statement usually does not exceed 5 percent. However, if the percentage is greater than 5, but less than 15, the survey conduct team must make one of two determinations. First, the team should determine whether the *strongly disagree* responses are simply a reflection of a pattern of strong disagreement in a particular department or in an unidentified segment of the organization. Second, the team should note in the survey action plan the strong disagreement with this statement and ask the human resources department to determine why the employees perceive lack of training and development opportunities. In this case, the basic action plan is for the human resources department to conduct a thorough training and development needs analysis survey to determine (1) whether the needs are real and (2) what those specific needs are.

Item 3

I understand how my job fits into the organization's "big picture" and the importance of what I do on a daily basis.

Item's Intent: To assess the employees' identification as being part of the efforts of the organization as a whole to provide high-quality health care on a daily basis.

Response Indicators and Action Plans:

SA Strong agreement with this statement should be at least 30 percent, because most health care employees are motivated by the fact that their jobs help to provide high-quality health care to the customer/patients. An employee's lack of recognition of his or her particular role in the overall provision of health care usually reflects the individual's problem with self-motivation.

A Agreement with this statement is usually 50 percent or more. Even if an individual does not agree with many of the items in the survey or feels that the organization has been somewhat lax in terms of meeting his or her own professional needs, he or she still has a strong sense of personal mission and of the importance of his or her job with the overall organizational mission.

N Neutral response to this statement usually does not exceed 10 percent. Most individuals either do or do not know how their job role fits into the organization's mission overall. Employees with limited interest in considering how their specific job fits into the organization's mission may select the *neutral* category because this issue is not an important factor in their daily motivation.

D Disagreement with this statement usually does not exceed 10 percent. If it does, there are two potential reasons why. First, an individual who responds negatively to this statement may feel that the organization is responsible for explaining to him or her just what the big picture is. In other words, the employee feels that the organization does a poor job of identifying its mission and its future goals. Usually, there is further comment about this in the comments and suggestions section, as well as similar response in section I (the Organization), where the organization's mission and its growth plans are discussed. If not, this response can be interpreted as inconsistent.

    Second, the individual does not understand that his or her job *does* affect the organization overall. A typical example of this is, "I work in accounting, therefore, I have very little to do with patient care." Obviously, this individual has not been educated properly by his or her manager about the relevance of his or her job to the organization overall. The action plan for this type of response is for the managers throughout the organization to emphasize to each employee the importance of his or her job to the overall success of the organization.

SD In many stellar health care organizations, strong disagreement with this statement is 0 percent. Most individuals, even nonplayers, know how their job relates to the big picture. If they do not, it is their fault. Strong disagreement with this statement indicates that the individual does not have a clue why he or she is employed. If, through performance evaluations and other measurable documentation, this individual is identified as a nonplayer, he or she should be educated immediately in no uncertain terms about the importance of his or her job. In essence, strong disagreement with this statement is a significant breach in allegiance to the organization.

Item 4

The relationship between the people in my department and the medical staff is relatively positive.

Item's Intent: To assess the employees' perception of the relationship among respondents, their respective departments, and the medical staff.

Response Indicators and Action Plans:

SA Strong agreement with this statement, usually generated by individuals who work closely with the medical staff, registers between 15 to 30 percent. The percentage range is large because the statement can be applicable or not, depending on the individual's job. It is important to look at the written comments and suggestions section because most individuals elaborate on this statement.

A In progressive health care organizations, agreement with this statement is between 45 to 60 percent. Even if an individual has limited exposure to physicians and other members of the medical staff, he or she believes that the relationship between them is relatively positive. It is a positive indicator if the organization receives an overall response rate exceeding 70 percent inclusive of the *agree* and *strongly agree* categories. Such a response rate should be publicized throughout the organization.

N Neutral response to this statement of 10 to 20 percent is not unusual. The foremost reason for neutral response is that the respondent has very little interaction with the medical staff. Therefore, neutral responses are not analyzed too thoroughly.

D Disagreement with this statement (10 to 20 percent) is usually generated by individuals who have a lot of interaction with the medical staff and feel that that interaction is often negative. Disagreement of less than 10 percent is a nonissue, merely reflecting some respondents' chronic negativity (as previously discussed) throughout this survey. However, if the response rate in the *disagree* category exceeds 10 percent, there is probably a problem with a particular physician or with physicians in general. In this case, three basic action plans should be implemented:

- Hold a discussion with the executive management staff and the physicians to determine whether there is a specific problem.
- Utilize as many specific comments and suggestions from the survey as possible in an effort to improve employee–physician relations.
- Survey physicians along with the individuals who indicated dissatisfaction with the physicians using specific survey methods. The survey results should be incorporated into an organizational development plan to improve employee–physician relations.

SD Strong disagreement with this statement usually does not exceed more than 5 percent. However, if 5 percent or more is registered, the action plans discussed in the *disagree* category should be implemented immediately.

Item 5

My job description adequately reflects 60 to 80 percent of my job and its regular ongoing responsibilities.

Item's Intent: To determine whether a majority of employees' ongoing responsibilities are fully reflected in their job descriptions. Most industrial psychologists agree that a job description honestly reflecting 60 to 100 percent of an individual's ongoing responsibilities is solidly constructed. If a job description is not sufficiently comprehensive, it can be misrepresentative and can be a negative motivator.

Response Indicators and Action Plans:

SA Strong agreement with this statement (20 to 30 percent) usually registers in organizations that have done a good job in terms of their total human resources management. In these organizations, employees have participated in constructing their job descriptions, which the managers have then ratified and continually updated.

A Agreement with this statement exceeds 50 percent in most progressive health care organizations. Once again, this is because employees have taken part in devising their job descriptions and feel comfortable with their content and comprehensiveness.

N Neutral response to this statement usually does not exceed 7 percent because by its nature the statement is a yes or no proposition. The only reason an employee is neutral regarding this statement is he or she does not know or care whether his or her job description is adequate.

D Disagreement with this statement usually does not exceed 10 percent. If it does, however, there are four action plans that the survey conduct team (in conjunction with the human resources department) can undertake:
- Review job descriptions and include the last date that the descriptions were revised.

- Determine whether the job descriptions are up-to-date and adequately reflect the jobs' responsibilities.
- Make employees aware of the fact that many job descriptions do not reflect more than 80 percent of the individual's ongoing responsibilities. However, many employees feel that the job description should reflect 100 percent of their job responsibilities. This is not a realistic possibility.
- Encourage employees to participate with managers in rewriting and updating job descriptions. This is particularly important in light of the requirements of the Americans with Disabilities Act and other crucial health care organizational dynamics.

SD Strong disagreement with this statement in excess of 5 percent is analyzed in conjunction with the action plans and recommendations in the *disagree* category. However, when an individual who registers strong disagreement with this statement volunteers his or her name and job position, the human resources department and/or the department manager should address the individual's problem specifically and promptly.

Item 6

I usually have the opportunity to give input and recommendations regarding my job activity.

Item's Intent: To determine the perceived amount of input the employees are allowed and encouraged to give on a daily basis.

Response Indicators and Action Plans:

SA Response to this statement is very subjective because employees have different ideas about what constitutes an appropriate amount of input. Strong agreement with this statement (exceeding 20 percent) in most good organizations is usually from individuals who are professionals who daily provide their manager with a significant amount of input. Additionally, some individuals feel they always have the opportunity to provide input, whether they take advantage of that opportunity or not.

Some employees are never satisfied with the amount of input they are allowed to give. Some jobs require providing more input (such as that of a surgeon or a highly skilled staff technician), and others require or need relatively little (such as a cafeteria worker or a medical records clerk). These issues are considered when analyzing all categories of response to this statement.

A Again, because of the subjective nature of this statement, agreement in the range of 40 to 60 percent is considered acceptable. A majority response in the two positive categories—*strongly agree* and *agree*—is a clear indicator that the organization utilizes an effective, practical form of participatory management.

N Neutral response to this statement indicates either apathy or indifference on the part of the individual. That is, the individual does not care whether he or she is allowed to give input. Such an individual simply wants to know what the job is, the salary, and the critical performance deadlines. Beyond those criteria, he or she has little interest in the job.

D Disagreement with this statement is usually less than 10 percent. When the response in the *disagree* category exceeds 10 percent, the possibility exists that a dictatorial form of management has taken root or that the employees, in general, are not satisfied with the amount of input they do have. Three reasons for disagreement with this statement are:

- The individual *believes* that he or she should be allowed to give more input.
- The individual feels that although he or she gives a certain amount of input, the manager does not follow his or her advice or follow it in a manner favorable to the respondent.
- The individual truly is not given an opportunity to provide input because the manager believes that the manager is the expert on the job.

   This last rationale is the only one that should be acted on by the survey conduct team. It is hoped that the individual has expanded on these feelings in the comments and suggestions section or elsewhere in the survey. An action plan in this case could include:

- Exploration of the management style used in certain areas of the organization
- Further discussion in employee–management forums and through other communication channels of the employees' feelings that they lack opportunity to provide input about their jobs

SD Strong disagreement with this statement rarely exceeds 5 percent. When it does, the same action plans suggested in the *disagree* category should be utilized. It is important to note that many individuals who strongly disagree with this statement are disgruntled employees in general. Therefore the survey conduct team should look for a pattern of negative responses throughout the survey and then deal with the individual employee, his or her manager, and/or human resources staff, if appropriate.

Item 7

Quality is vital to my job performance and work output.

Item's Intent: To assess the employees' perception of the importance of quality in conducting their daily responsibilities.

Response Indicators and Action Plans:

SA Of all of the statements in section 3, this one usually draws the highest percentage of strong agreement (50 percent or more) for two reasons. First, many individuals in health care organizations have been exposed to the quality improvement movement in American health care and consider themselves to be advocates of that process. Second, many health care employees recognize the importance of quality outcomes, particularly in respect to the potential impact on the quality of life and health of the customer/patient. Therefore, even the most malevolent and disloyal employees register a strong amount of agreement relative to their own personal quest for quality in their job roles.

A Agreement with this statement also runs high (25 percent or more), although proportionately less than in the *strongly agree* category. The reasons for agreement are identical to those described in the *strongly agree* category.

N Neutral response to this statement is usually never more than 4 percent, the reason being that individuals are well aware of quality and recognize that their pursuit of quality is essential to job success. Therefore, it is rare that individuals select the *neutral* category in response to this statement.

D Disagreement with this statement usually does not exceed 10 percent. However, if it is in excess of 10 percent, an investigation is launched to determine why these individuals feel that quality is not an important part of their jobs. Employee disagreement is rooted in three causes:

- The organization has not undertaken continuous quality improvement (CQI) as an organizational initiative.
- The organization has not encouraged individuals to achieve quality as part of their daily process.
- The individual feels that managers (particularly his or her supervisor) do not allow him or her to pursue quality. Or, the individual feels that the manager acts as a barrier to the employee's achievement of quality results. In this case, a close review of the same respondent's section on management, and particularly statements related to his or her manager, are examined to ascertain a cause or pattern. However, further examination of this problem can be difficult when the individual has not identified himself or herself.

SD Strong disagreement with this statement is usually no more than 5 percent. However, if response in the *strongly disagree* category exceeds 5 percent, the same investigative technique suggested in the *disagree* category should be used.

Item 8

There are solid opportunities in the organization to grow in my particular area of expertise.

Item's Intent: To determine employees' perceptions of opportunities to enhance their careers and professional growth.

Response Indicators and Action Plans:

SA Strong agreement with this statement (10 percent or more) indicates that the top echelon of employee performers feel that they have the opportunity to achieve and grow within the organization. This sentiment is enhanced by employee development programs and individual development plans as part of the human resources strategic process.

A Agreement with this statement is as high as 40 percent in stellar health care organizations. In sound health care organizations, a response rate of 25 percent or more in the *agree* category is satisfactory, indicating that individuals recognize that they have opportunities (such as promotions and job enhancement programs) to grow within the organization. Furthermore, individuals who respond positively to this statement usually have enjoyed some sort of promotion or job expansion opportunity during their tenure at the organization.

N Neutral response to this statement (particularly if it exceeds 20 percent) may indicate any of four organizational dynamics. First, some individuals equate growth opportunities strictly with promotion. Because many health care organizations are not constantly growing, some employees are frustrated at the lack of opportunities for vertical job movement.

Second, some employees fail to see the opportunity to enhance their jobs by expanding their responsibilities. They become demotivated because they do not believe they have the opportunity to enrich their job scope or take on new opportunities.

Third, some employees feel that growth opportunities are strictly measured by increased compensation. Although increased compensation for increased responsibilities is ideal, it is difficult for some individuals to stay motivated when they have been assigned additional responsibility but no additional compensation. Unfortunately, this situation is a reality in many health care organizations where most employees are told to "do more with less."

Fourth, some employees are not interested in growth opportunities. They feel they are well placed in their current job and do not desire or need any growth opportunities.

Action plans the organization can utilize to counteract *neutral* or even *disagree* responses to this statement include these:

- The organization should clearly identify career paths and promotional opportunities for each particular job. This task is largely the responsibility of the human resources department, but the effort must be supported by every line manager and supervisor within the organization.
- Managers should take the responsibility to have frank discussions with their employees to let them know that there are limited promotional opportunities within the organization.
- The organization should utilize the concepts of job expansion and enrichment, supplemented by appropriate compensation strategies when possible.
- Under no condition or in any situation should a manager provide false hope to any employee relative to a job opportunity or promotional situation that will never occur.

D   In most organizations, disagreement with this statement is less than 20 percent. Individuals' reasons for disagreement are the same as for those who selected the *neutral* category but voiced with more negativity. That is, the respondent wants the organization to know that he or she not only sees no growth opportunities, but is angry about the situation. Again, incorporating the concepts of job enrichment and job expansion into the organization are important factors in addressing negative responses to this statement.

SD Strong disagreement with this statement does not usually exceed 10 percent. However, if responses to this statement vary from being in the *neutral* to the *strongly disagree* categories, the organization must take a serious look at job opportunities organizationwide. A problem might be the hiring of new employees after failing to promote individuals from within the organization. This problem can be remedied by immediately implementing a strong development and internal promotion/posting program.

Item 9

My current job provides me with a reasonable degree of professional fulfillment and career satisfaction.

Item's Intent: To assess the employees' perception of individual job satisfaction.

Response Indicators and Action Plans:

SA Strong agreement with this statement is usually 30 percent or more. Fundamentally, if individuals were not satisfied with their current responsibilities, they would leave the organization in search of better job situations.

A Agreement (usually 40 percent or more) is often the most common response to this statement. Again, this response is due to individual perception. Some individuals are satisfied with their jobs, while others in the exact same positions are dissatisfied. Because there are a variety or reasons why individuals are or are not satisfied, it is important to consider any comments or suggestions that further discuss response to this statement.

N Neutral response to this statement is usually not more than 10 percent because individuals have strong opinions about whether they are satisfied with their current jobs. The nature of the statement calls for a yes or no answer. Details about responses to this question are often provided in the comments and suggestions section of the survey.

D Disagreement with this statement does not usually exceed 15 percent. The turnover figure among health care professionals nationally is slightly in excess of 15 percent. Therefore, the survey conduct team can compare the *disagree* category's rate of response with the turnover figure the organization registered in the previous calendar year. Usually, these percentages are within three points of each other.

   If an individual disagrees or strongly disagrees with the statement that he or she is satisfied with his or her current job, the survey reviewer should take a close look at the comments and suggestions provided at the bottom of the page. As previously stated, this disagreement could be another example of a chronic complaint. Unfortunately, such complainers will seldom identify themselves, not out of fear of reprisal, but because they are using the survey to play a "mind game." In most organizations, managers have a good idea of which employees are satisfied with their work roles. It is hoped that the managers have taken steps to ensure that only the satisfied, motivated individuals remain with the organization.

SD Strong disagreement with this statement rarely exceeds 2 percent. If someone is very dissatisfied, it is only logical to assume that he or she has sought or is in the process of seeking other employment. In some cases, if an individual who selects the *strongly disagree* category in response to this statement identifies himself or herself, he or she may be asking for help in "sorting out" personal feelings in regard to his or her professional role. In this case, the manager should seize the opportunity to forthrightly and fully discuss these sentiments with the employee.

Item 10

Overall, I am motivated and interested in my job, my career, and the contribution I make to the organization.

Item's Intent: To determine the amount of motivation employees bring to work every day.

Response Indicators and Action Plans:

SA Strong agreement with this statement is usually 45 percent or more because, as a group, health care professionals are usually motivated by a set of personal factors (such as work and personal ethics). Consequently, most organizations register a large response in this category.

A Agreement with this statement is also usually large. At a combined rate of 75 to 85 percent, responses in the *strongly agree* and *agree* categories usually comprise the overwhelming response to the statement. Again, most health care employees are motivated and will discount minor negatives in considering their overall motivation.

N The neutral responses to this statement are very important to look at. If an individual selects the *neutral* category and if an overall neutral response rate of 5 percent or more is registered, the organization should assess how recent events and/or other organizational dynamics may be hampering employee motivation.

D Disagreement with this statement greater than 10 percent must be examined closely by executive management. In this case, it is vital to determine the various causes for lack of motivation among employees. Recent change, negative financial results, and a host of other organizationally related factors may contribute to this problem.

SD Strong disagreement of 5 percent or more with this statement is investigated closely by the executive management group. Strong disagreement may focus on the individual, the department, the organization, or in some cases, the overall environment. It is important to remember that motivation is an individual dynamic and (as previously stated) lack of motivation may indicate an individual who is currently looking for employment elsewhere or who should be. Responses in the *strongly disagree* category are compared with other responses throughout the survey to determine any patterns and trends in the responses.

    An important factor among employees who register strong disagreement with this statement is the belief that motivation is not their personal responsibility. They feel it is the organization's responsibility to motivate them (through additional compensation, for example). In the real world, every adult is responsible for his or her own actions. Therefore, certain responses to this statement in the *strongly disagree* category should be taken with a grain of salt and not overanalyzed by the survey conduct team.

Analysis Guide Section IV:
The Work Environment/General Issues

Item 1

Our organization is "people-oriented," that is, genuinely concerned about patients and employees.

Item's Intent: To determine employees' perception on how people-oriented the organization is on a daily basis.

Response Indicators and Action Plans:

SA Strong agreement with this statement of 25 percent or more is outstanding, indicating that most respondents believe their organization is consciously directed toward providing a people-oriented delivery system to its customer/patients.

A Agreement with this statement is usually 50 percent or more in strong health care organizations. Agreement is usually the more popular response to this statement because many individuals are able to cite an area in which people-oriented customer service could be increased. There is always room for improvement in the delivery of health care services.

N Neutral response to this statement is typically 10 to 20 percent in most good health care organizations. Neutral responses may indicate that respondents are not directly involved in customer/patient relations. Accordingly, they feel that they do not have significant knowledge to respond to this statement. Additionally, many individuals may select the *neutral* category if they believe that the organization is satisfactorily providing people-oriented customer service.

D Disagreement with this statement at 20 percent or more is a red flag for any health care organization, indicating that a fifth of the employees feel the customer/patients are not receiving the appropriate people-oriented service. In this case, three action plans should be considered:
- The organization could implement a customer service program to educate all organization members about the importance of strong customer/patient relations.
- Specific employee focus groups could be organized and meetings conducted to identify specific areas in which the organization should improve its customer/patient relations. Examples of poor customer service should be defined, evidence of poor customer service should be presented by focus group members, and, most important, solutions to improve customer relations should be discussed.
- Managers could take an active role in discussing customer/patient relations with their employees in an informal manner (for example, during

working hours and within the context of weekly meetings). These discussions should highlight specific ways individual employees can contribute to stronger customer relations in the delivery of health care services.

SD Strong disagreement with this statement usually does not exceed 5 percent. If it does, however, the organization should consider utilizing the strategies outlined in the *disagree* category. If the response rate in the *strongly disagree* category exceeds 10 percent, the organization should *immediately* implement those action strategies.

Item 2

Most of the people who work here are dedicated and motivated to provide high-quality health care.

Item's Intent: To assess the employees' dedication to the mission and objectives of the health care organization in providing high-quality health care.

Response Indicators and Action Plans:

SA Strong agreement with this statement is typically 25 to 35 percent because many employees recognize that the majority of their coworkers are dedicated to the hospital's mission as evidenced in their everyday activities. Many employees also recognize superior examples of dedication to the organization's mission.

A Agreement with this statement is usually 50 percent or more because many employees are quick to recognize their own and coworkers' dedication to their particular jobs and to the larger organization's mission.

N Neutral response to this statement is usually less than 10 percent because many employees clearly understand the statement, its intent, and the impact of employee dedication on the overall organizational environment. In this case, response in the *neutral* category must be interpreted as a satisfactory response.

D Disagreement with this statement is usually less than 10 percent (and less than 5 percent in many organizations). If disagreement with this statement is 10 percent or more, the response may indicate a lack of employee morale organizationwide. Fundamentally, if individuals are not dedicated to the basic mission of the organization, they are not dedicated to the mission of health care.

SD Strong disagreement with this statement usually does not exceed 5 percent. If it does, the survey analysis team must recognize that a problem with employee morale exists. Morale problems are then more clearly identified by examining other responses in this section and throughout the survey generally.

Item 3

Most of the people I work with "know their stuff," have a good degree of expertise, and are up-to-date in their field.

Item's Intent: To assess the perceived level of staff expertise organizationwide.

Response Indicators and Action Plans:

SA Strong agreement with this statement exceeds 25 percent in most good organizations. Most health care employees realize that their specific technical responsibilities mandate a high level of expertise. Furthermore, with the help and encouragement of the organization, employees are expected to stay up-to-date in their field. This process requires employees to pursue continuing education opportunities, to incorporate new technologies, and to master new approaches and methods for providing health care.

A Agreement with this statement is usually 50 percent or more in most strong health care organizations and it is not uncommon to see the rate exceed 60 percent in some stellar health care organizations. Most health care employees recognize that they are responsible for maintaining their own level of expertise. Accordingly, they will give themselves high marks in this regard. Organizations registering well with this statement in the *strongly agree* and/or *agree* categories are usually utilizing the following four strategies:

- They have a well-established professional development program, augmented by ongoing technical education in various fields.
- They have an ongoing series of on-site, in-service educational programs that provide new technical education.
- They have a commitment from the executive management group, supported by the actions of all managers and supervisors, to promote educational opportunities for employees both at the institution and off-site (such as at local community colleges and by professional organizations).
- They are committed to providing proper funding and other types of support necessary for education at all levels.

      The organization that provides opportunities to enhance technical expertise is one that will not only prosper but will engender a strong sense of trust, pride, and morale among employees. This issue must merit special attention from the survey conduct team and the health care organization's executive management group.

N Neutral response to this statement is usually less than 7 percent, even if the majority of respondents disagree with this statement. This is because the statement is basically a yes or no proposition. Either the organization has individuals who "know their stuff" or it does not. Therefore, individuals will have a strong opinion one way or the other to this statement.

D   Disagreement with this statement does not exceed 10 percent in a strong health care organization. If it does, two problems may be the cause. First, there may be a lack of continuing education opportunities provided by the organization to all employees. This situation can be remedied by adopting the four strategies outlined in the *agree* category.

Second, there may be problems in the hiring and selection process for new employees that allow managers to choose individuals who are not of the highest professional caliber. If this statement receives a *disagree* or *strongly disagree* rating that exceeds 10 percent, the organization must pursue two action plans:

- Executive management tries to elicit specific examples of employees who are perceived as "not knowing their stuff." This is a tricky process. It is difficult for employees to identify other employees without feeling as though their confidentiality is being threatened. It is therefore incumbent upon the managers to determine whether there is a lack of adequate employee expertise.
- The organization creates a structured hiring system to help screen qualified applicants. Quality health care organizations use several hiring methods.

SD   Strong disagreement with this statement usually does not exceed 5 percent. However, if it does, it must be considered in conjunction with the response rate in the *disagree* category. In this case, the action plans outlined in the *disagree* category must be pursued immediately.

Item 4

Most of the people I work with are proud of our organization and believe in its goals, objectives, and philosophies.

Item's Intent: To assess employees' collective pride throughout the organization relative to the organization's actions and goals.

Response Indicators and Action Plans:

SA   Although the presence of a collective pride in the organization is paramount to a health care organization's success, strong agreement with this statement usually does not exceed 15 percent. It should be noted that a collective sense of pride is never 100 percent in any organization owing to various events. For example, a current reality in many American health care institutions is downsizing. When employees get laid off, it is difficult for the remaining employees (even in a strong organization) to feel proud. The response rate in the *agree* category provides a more accurate reflection of the level of employee pride.

A   In a strong health care organization, agreement with this statement usually exceeds 50 percent. This statement is basically a yes or no proposition.

That is, individuals either feel a strong sense of allegiance to the organization or they do not. It is difficult for employees to disagree with this statement, unless there is a prevailing sense of low morale or they are affected by an issue that is currently causing resentment.

N   A neutral response rate to this statement is proportionately more than to other statements. It is not uncommon for it to be 20 percent or more, and the survey conduct team should interpret this rate as satisfactory. That is, most individuals feel that they and their colleagues are relatively proud of the organization and believe in its goals and objectives. Additionally, a large response in the *neutral* category reflects the feelings of the steady players, most of whom are not motivated by a strong sense of pride. They merely want a steady paycheck and clear direction in performing their jobs.

D   Disagreement with this statement usually does not exceed 10 percent. If it does, the organization has a problem with employee allegiance to its goals and mission. To correct this problem, the organization should undertake three basic action plans:
   • The organization should implement various development strategies to increase the motivation of individuals throughout the organization.
   • The organization should assess the effect of any major crisis or negative events (such as massive layoffs, freezing or hiring, or lack of pay raises).
   • The organization should determine whether its mission and goals have been clearly articulated to all members of the organization.

SD Strong disagreement with this statement usually does not exceed 5 percent. If it does, the survey conduct team should alert the executive management group to this fact. The team should also consider the response percentage in the *strongly disagree* category in concert with other responses throughout the survey relative to motivation, morale, and allegiance.

Item 5

Most of my colleagues are relatively motivated and satisfied with the organization and their work roles.

Item's Intent: To determine the level of morale generated by the employees in their daily work lives throughout the organization.

Response Indicators and Action Plans:

SA Strong agreement with this statement usually does not exceed 10 percent. Employee morale is either present or not. With all the ongoing changes in health care (including government intervention and regulatory mandates), employee morale does not often register in the *strongly agree* category. Furthermore, individuals in different areas of the country have different reactions to this statement. For example, in some rural areas employee morale is higher than in certain urban areas. In the Midwest, ratings are a little higher than on either coast. Once again, external economic factors play a part in responses to this statement.

A Agreement with this statement is usually the stronger response. In a good organization, agreement in excess of 50 percent indicates high employee morale. Any response in the *agree* category between 40 to 60 percent is considered a positive indicator to this statement.

N In a good organization, neutral response to this statement is usually between 20 and 30 percent. Individuals select the *neutral* category for two reasons; either as a satisfactory rating or as an "I don't care about this" response. Some individuals feel their morale is "O.K." as long as they are getting adequate compensation.

D Disagreement with this statement is usually less than 20 percent. A response rate greater than 20 percent indicates a current negative situation or a recent negative situation that angered the entire organization. It may also indicate a prevailing feeling of negative morale due to a compensation issue. In this case, the survey conduct team must look at specific incidences in the organization's recent history to determine how the *disagree* category percentage may be reflecting feelings toward a specific organizational dynamic.

SD Strong disagreement with this statement usually does not exceed 3 percent. Although many individuals may have a negative reaction to the employee morale issue, they will not select the *strongly disagree* category unless a central, significant issue is being contended. Significant issues include:
- A union campaign
- A recent layoff
- A freeze on wage increases
- A merger or acquisition
- A negative environmental factor, such as the closing of a major local employer

These factors should be identified and their impact on the organization objectively presented to all employees in the postsurvey briefing meetings. In these meetings, employees should be asked why they think morale is low. The organization must utilize employee responses to construct an action plan that will resolve problems to employee morale.

Item 6

My pay level is fair considering my job role.

Item's Intent: To determine whether employees feel that their compensation level is fair in comparison with standard market rates and other factors relative to health care compensation.

Response Indicators and Action Plans:

SA   Strong agreement with this statement never exceeds 10 percent. Most individuals in health care know how their compensation levels rate compared to market standards. Accordingly, they can make a clear-cut determination on whether they are being paid fairly and are very vocal in registering their opinions on this matter. In many cases, if there is an issue relative to compensation (or perceived unfair compensation), it will be highlighted prior to the survey and addressed subsequently.

A   Agreement with this statement is usually 50 percent or more because most health care organizations are diligent about conducting wage surveys on a regular basis. Because they are aware of a health care organization's financial limitations due to the current economic climate and other factors, most health care employees have realistic expectations relative to their compensation level. If their expectations are being met, this statement is not an issue for them.

N   Neutral response to this statement registered at 15 percent or less, indicates that employees are basically satisfied with their level of compensation. If an individual is not satisfied, he or she utilizes one of the *disagree* categories.

D   Disagreement with this statement is usually less than 25 percent. Although this percentage is proportionately higher than other negative percentages throughout the survey, the survey conduct team must keep in mind that most individuals feel their compensation level should be higher. (They can always point to another organization that pays a higher rate for a similar job.)

    If there is a response in the *strongly disagree* category of more than 25 percent, the organization should undertake five action plans:

- A wage survey that illustrates pay norms throughout the operating region should be conducted immediately.
- A study should be conducted by the human resources department to determine whether the amount of pay raises and the frequency of pay adjustments is commensurate with market norms throughout the area.
- The organization should highlight compensation package benefits other than financial, so that the employees fully recognize that their paycheck is only one part of the compensation package.
- Any economic conditions (such as shrinking operating budgets, for example) should be presented to the employees forthrightly and clearly in order that they understand the organization's limitations relative to financial remuneration.

- The organization should make the case that its pay structure is in the top 25 percent, if not the top 50 percent, of all health care organizations in the region. The organization should pay at a rate that is at least higher than the median average wage for a particular job in that area. For example, if most staff nurses in Wyoming make $35,000 a year and if a particular Wyoming hospital's pay for staff nurses is less than $35,000, its employees have a legitimate gripe relative to this statement.

SD Strong disagreement with this statement usually does not exceed 5 percent. If it does, the organization should immediately investigate whether compensation dissatisfaction exists in several departments, within a technical area, or organizationwide. Wage surveys and other investigative measures should be taken to ensure that employee turnover is not exacerbated by a problem with employee compensation.

Item 7

Mediocre/marginal performance is not tolerated within the organization.

Item's Intent: To assess whether negative performance on the part of employees is tolerated.

Response Indicators and Action Plans:

SA Strong agreement with this statement is usually 25 percent or more. That is, many individuals in a premier organization feel that negative performers are dealt with appropriately.

A Agreement with this statement usually exceeds 50 percent. If response in the *agree* category is less than 50 percent there is a problem. In fact, if the response rate in the *agree* category combined with the response rate in the *strongly agree* category is less than 60 percent, there is cause for alarm. Poor performance in health care is easily recognized by both employees and managers. In seminars conducted by the author, most individuals indicated that they can recognize the poor performance of a colleague within a two-week period. However, the manager might take longer to recognize such performance. And due to legal and organizational regulations, the manager can take even longer to address the poor performance through performance evaluation or dismissal. It is critical to employee morale that negative performers are not tolerated.

N Neutral response to this statement of 15 percent or less is usual in most good health care organizations because the employee may not yet have considered this issue as thoroughly or thoughtfully as he or she might have considered others addressed by the survey.

D Disagreement with this statement of 15 percent or more indicates that negative performers might be tolerated either organizationwide or in selective departments. As any health care manager knows, there are short-ages in many technical areas, including nursing, physical therapy, and pharmacy. Therefore, some managers are hesitant to dismiss an employee for fear of not being able to find a suitable replacement. As a result, many individuals are retained, although their performance levels and motivation are suspect in the eyes of their coworkers.

An organization that receives a response rate in the *disagree* category exceeding 15 percent should examine its performance evaluation sys-tem. Furthermore, the executive leadership of the organization should encourage all managers and supervisors to make strides in document-ing performance and addressing negative performance appropriately. This mandate must come from top management and extend down throughout the organization.

SD Strong disagreement with this statement usually does not exceed 5 per-cent. If it does, there is usually one specific employee group in which a number of negative performers have been allowed to work without reprisal or negative consequence. Whenever possible, the survey con-duct team should identify such pockets of negative performance and address the problem with the manager in charge.

Item 8

If a conflict arises on the job between my manager and myself, there are ways available in the organization for a resolution.

Item's Intent: To determine whether conflicts between managers and employees are resolved quickly and that certain organizational methods are in place to facilitate conflict management.

Response Indicators and Action Plans:

SA Strong agreement with this statement at 10 percent or more is excellent, indicating that there is a general perception on the part of the employees that conflict is resolved quickly and in an appropriate manner. This state-ment does not generate a large percentage in the *strongly agree* category unless the respondent was personally involved in a situation where the organization took steps to resolve a conflict positively and in his or her favor. In other words, the conflict turned out the way that the respon-dent hoped it would.

A   The agreement response rate is a more accurate reflection of the employees' perception of conflict resolution strategies. In most health care organizations, a response rate of 50 percent or more in the *agree* category is positive, indicating a general acknowledgment of the exis-tence of conflict resolution strategies throughout the organization and a commitment from most, if not all, managers to resolve conflict quickly and positively.

N A neutral response of 15 to 25 percent is considered the norm in most health care organizations because neutral responses may simply indicate that the individual has never had the opportunity or need for conflict resolution.

D Disagreement with this statement at 20 percent or more indicates that, in the estimation of the employees, conflict is not being resolved properly. Three reasons for disagreement with this statement include:

- The feeling on the part of employees that managers avoid confronting conflict because they lack the fortitude to deal with it.
- Individuals throughout the organization create and claim their own "turf," creating a divisive atmosphere.
- Certain managers and employees generate conflict intentionally.

The result of such disharmonious sentiments could be a union organization campaign, wide-scale employee dissatisfaction, or a mass exodus of good employees who leave for other organizations. Action plans to counteract the percentages in the *disagree* category include the following:

- The organization should employ a chain-of-command policy in which conflict is resolved by managers progressively up the chain of command until conflict is resolved.
- The organization should provide training for all managers in resolving conflict.
- The organization should discourage any turf claiming or elitist attitudes among employees.
- The organization's leadership should ensure that all managers know how to resolve conflict and how to deal promptly and properly with individuals who generate conflict, particularly if they are poor performers.

SD Strong disagreement with this statement usually does not exceed 5 percent. A response rate of 10 percent or less in the *strongly disagree* category usually indicates a situation wherein the individuals who started conflicts saw the outcomes go in their favor. However, any strong disagreement exceeding 10 percent must be reviewed with the responses in the *disagree* category. If the combined percentages of these two categories indicate a dissatisfaction with conflict resolution organizationwide, the executive leadership should take the four actions prescribed in the *disagree* category.

Item 9

Generally speaking, most work efforts at our organization are pursued in a quality-conscious, cost-effective manner.

Item's Intent: To determine employees' assessment of the organization's ability to provide health care services and products in a quality conscious, cost-effective manner.

Response Indicators and Action Plans:

SA Strong agreement with this statement at 10 percent or more is a positive indicator that the quality control initiatives taken by the organization are effective. Most organizations feel that all members of the organization should have an awareness of quality initiatives, and thus the response to this statement is very important.

A Agreement is typically the strongest response indicated in most organizations. A good rate of agreement with this statement is 55 percent or more. Because most health care members are inundated by quality improvement literature and related programs, they may have become numb to quality platitudes. Therefore, most will agree with this statement, but not get too excited with its premise. It is hoped that individuals recognize the link between cost-effectiveness and quality, and consider the statement accordingly.

N Neutral response to this statement may be 20 percent or more. Many individuals mark neutral because they feel that although they are quality conscious personally, they do not know about the rest of the organization. Some organizations insert the phrase "to the best of my knowledge" in the statement. As it stands, however, the statement will elicit an indication of employees' perception of the success of quality initiatives in the organization. If an individual feels that provision of quality is not a standard throughout the organization or that limited finances are being squandered owing to a lack of cost-effectiveness, he or she will *not* have a neutral response to this statement. Rather, the respondent will select the *disagree* or *strongly disagree* category. Therefore, it is the author's contention that this statement is valid as it stands and that neutral response to it indicates mild agreement.

D Disagreement with this statement usually does not exceed 12 percent. If it does, the survey conduct team must make two determinations. First, they should determine whether the disagreement is centered in one particular department. Second, they should conduct a second survey of the individuals involved in the quality process to elicit specific examples of a lack of quality or cost-effectiveness.

SD Strong disagreement with this statement is usually never higher than 5 percent. If it is, the survey conduct team should conduct further surveys and utilize other investigative techniques to uncover the specific areas lacking in quality and/or cost-effectiveness.

Item 10

Considering my employment status, the organization provides a satisfactory benefits package.

Item's Intent: To assess the employees' satisfaction whatever their employment status (part-time or full-time, for example) relative to the current benefits package.

Response Indicators and Action Plans:

SA Strong agreement with this statement usually never exceeds 10 percent. Most employees recognize that health benefits have soaring costs attached to them. Therefore, they are somewhat skeptical about their organization's ability to provide a good benefits package. Furthermore, benefits packages offered by health care institutions in the United States are shrinking, and so a strong agreement response with this statement is uncommon.

A Agreement with this statement exceeding 40 percent is excellent. Because benefits are shrinking and many employees desire additional benefits (such as adult day care, extended child care, dental benefits, and so on), this statement does not generate a large positive response. Therefore, if the organization achieves a response rate of 40 percent or more in the *agree* category, it is indeed doing something right relative to benefits administration.

N Neutral response to this statement typically ranges from 15 to 25 percent because many employees do not know what is fair relative to a benefits package. Therefore, they cannot agree or disagree with this statement. It is important for the survey conduct team to look very closely at the neutral response to this statement. If the response rate in the *neutral* category is particularly high (in excess of 20 percent), it is important for the organization's administration to make clear presentations to the employees relative to the benefits package and to proactively dispel any rumors by demonstrating the link between the general economy and the organization's ability to provide a comprehensive benefits package.

D Disagreement with this statement is usually between 20 and 35 percent because, as previously stated, most individuals desire more benefits and, in many cases, are not completely satisfied with their benefits package. If this statement elicits a response rate of 25 percent in the *disagree* category, the organization must take action. A questionnaire relative to specific employee benefit needs and wants should be circulated. The needs and wants discussed in the questionnaire should then be clearly and forthrightly addressed by the organization.

SD Strong disagreement with this statement usually never exceeds 10 percent. Because shrinking employment benefits are a fact in America today, individuals are thankful for any benefits they do receive. Strong disagreement is usually centered on the need of a particular employee to have a major benefit added to the package. However, if the *strongly disagree* category receives a response rate greater than 15 percent, the organization should take a closer look at its benefits package by asking the following three questions:

- Is the benefits package comparable to others in the regional operating area?
- Does the benefits package lack a particular benefit demanded or needed by most of the employees?
- Has the organization made a proper budgetary allotment for benefits provision?

It is important that the organization examine its benefits package on the basis of results of this survey. Benefits are more important than paychecks to most health care employees.

Appendix C

Supplemental Survey Items

Organizations may want to customize their surveys by substituting new items for those in the standard survey instrument (appendix A). These substitutions can be based on a specific need or management preference. This appendix contains 20 additional items that may prove useful to individual organizations. In customizing the survey, the following principles should be kept in mind:

1. No section should contain more than 10 items in total so that comments and suggestions remain pertinent and focused.
2. Any items that differ from the standard format should not use absolute words such as *always, never,* or *100 percent of the time.*
3. Any new items should be placed in the appropriate section in the survey.
4. All of the items should be formulated as statements and refer to specific organizational, management, or job dynamics.

Some additional items that may be substituted are these:

- Most employees feel that this organization is a good place to work and to develop their career so as to reach their professional goals.
- For the most part, senior management understands the challenges and demands of the work roles of most of the organization members.
- In my opinion, turnover and employee resignations are not based on poor working conditions or inferior pay scales.
- The managers in this organization usually "know their stuff" and are fair and capable leaders.
- There are a satisfactory number of educational and developmental programs in this organization that are helpful and meaningful.
- National health care reform is something that we will adjust to and handle in this organization.

- Most of my friends and neighbors in the community think that our organization is a high-quality, progressive health care provider.
- I envision a long-term and enjoyable work life here.
- Most of my peers and colleagues feel that, in general, this is a good place to work.
- There is no lack of equipment or technology that I need to perform my job fully and competently.
- From an organizationwide perspective, I would say that we are ready for the future.
- I have a good understanding of how the organization will grow and prosper in the near future.
- I have a good understanding of how the organization will grow and prosper in the long term.
- Most new employees receive good orientation and understand the direction and scope of the organization.
- The quality improvement programs instituted by the organization have been useful and meaningful to me.
- The existing performance evaluation process is comprehensible and fair.
- The benefits package provided by the organization is reasonable and provides me with a generally secure feeling.
- Termination and probation are used rightfully when an individual constantly displays poor performance.
- Most of the changes in this organization are positive and produce progressive results.
- The leadership of this organization is intelligent, capable, and in touch with the staff as well as the local community.

Appendix D

Sample Action Plan

The following example of an organizationwide action plan is based on the innovations of three leading health care organizations resulting from their use of the survey system described in this book. (The names of the institutions do not appear, and, in some cases, information has been altered to preserve the privacy of the organizations' survey results.)

Resultant Issues and Recommendations of the Organizational Study

Issue 1: Communication

Increased communication should be attempted in providing information regarding the organization's future—plans, long-term goals, and so on—as well as new policies, changes in policies, organizational decisions that affect all employees, project updates, and the rationale behind all major projects or programs. Additionally, consultants' contributions should be communicated effectively so that appropriate managers and employees can take advantage of opportunities for learning. Also, the need for specific expertise in certain cases should be communicated in such a manner that internal resources are considered before engaging outside resources.

Recommended Actions:

1. Increase scope of the newsletter to include "organizational updates" and similar profile education (that is, information about the organization, its plans, goals, and other relevant news).
2. Utilize "executive memorandum" system for all managers on applicable issues and projects.

3. Review all internal sources and ask technical specialists for recommendations prior to outside contracting.

Issue 2: Wages and Benefits

The survey, management meetings, and national recession together have sent a message that the organization's compensation system is perceived as needing improvement. Regarding compensation, wage surveys seem limited and "hard to sell." Benefits in general are under close scrutiny by employees, notably with respect to pension and day care.

Recommended Actions:

1. Display job description criteria, union/nonunion, wage adjudication, and other aspects of "comp packages" in future wage surveys.
2. Educate managers that certain employees will contest *any* wage data and thus should be managed accordingly.
3. Review as a team, with an eye toward directly addressing day care overcrowding in certain age groups, pharmacy, pension, medical insurance, and vacation benefits. Dental and eye care should also be discussed, particularly in a dialogue concerning possible "flex/menu" plans. Given the exorbitant cost of employee benefits, explanation of costs, national trends, and other dynamics should be communicated as appropriate.
4. The shift differential issue, sick day policy, and day care issue should be addressed directly, as per our discussion.

Issue 3: Management Feedback

Managers indicated that feedback could be improved from employee to manager, as well as from managers to executives. It also could be improved in the areas of organizational planning and current issues, management ideas and input, and specific technical issues, such as new equipment purchases, specific acumen, and other specialty area applications. Though not deemed by any participant as a hot issue, management feedback was still a source of concern to approximately 20 percent of the various management participation groups.

Recommended Actions:

1. Adopt the plan cited in issue 1.
2. Use participation groups quarterly (for example, a forum conducted during a management survey luncheon).
3. Conduct a survey on more specific issues in the coming year.

4. In general, underscore the themes of "keeping an open mind," "really listening," and "explaining why" as standards of daily management conduct.

Issue 4: Management Issues

"Employees and physicians hear about things before managers," "we have too much time wasted in poorly managed/unnecessary meetings," and "we realize we have to do more with less but want to be paid for it" are accurate paraphrases of the negative issues raised in the responses to this category. A positive issue—"the employee picnic was great/want more events like this"—was widely endorsed.

Recommended Actions

1. In some cases, employees and physicians might hear about things first because those issues pertain to them directly. In other cases, communication might be secondary to the need for swift action.
2. Regarding meetings, a "miniseminar" of two or three hours on meeting management would be beneficial.
3. If job enhancement/enrichment becomes part of the normal job conduct, a wage review might be in order or cited as part of the performance evaluation.

Issue 5: Education and Development

Training and development were acknowledged to be credible parts of our management equation, but some specific suggestions were made that denote the following recommendations.

Recommended Actions:

1. Educational programs should include on-site GED, literacy, and basic community college-level courses.
2. The management mentoring program should be "revitalized."
3. Program evaluation should be conducted on existing programs by the participants.
4. A "nonthreatening" needs analysis should be conducted for future organizational planning for training and development.

Issue 6: Performance Issues

Performance at all levels of the organization could be enhanced, in the estimation of the management team, by adopting the following strategies:

1. Avoid suffering from "paralysis by analysis," that is, too much deliberation.
2. *Truly* control and manage our allocated resources, trust each other, and increase and exemplify our areas of expertise.
3. Educate our employees on the organization's mission, national health care dynamics, technical expertise, and "self-management" of time and effort.
4. Explain to our employees the rationale of the new lobby: customer excellence, the organization's national competitive relevance, local competition, clientele demands, physician and employee recruitment, and plant development.

Issue 7: Performance Evaluation System

The entire organization is apparently dissatisfied with the current performance evaluation system. Immediate action should be taken to modify the current form and system with the following goals:

1. Recognize different levels of performance more critically and constructively.
2. Reward performance "above and beyond" the norm with criterion-based mechanics.
3. Incorporate aspects of sound documentation and other dynamics into related educational efforts.
4. Restore incentives for stellar performance and consequences for negative performance to the system without "blanket" or unsubstantiated scoring.
5. Renew managerial and employee confidence and credibility to the system.

Issue 8: "In My Opinion . . ."

Comments and suggestions provided by managerial staff:

1. "Union talk is just something used by malcontents when they're being counseled."
2. "Coffee time" with executive staff members would facilitate communication.
3. More education is needed for new managers in physician orientation and in management orientation, for secretaries and clerical workers, and on national health care issues that are relevant to us here.
4. Videos could be made to educate "us" on construction projects, organizational events and issues, and other "timely topics."
5. In-house selection system is unfair/ineffective (canard or fact?).
6. The organization's "original" mission is diluted (−) or changing (+).
7. Lecture/meeting facility will be needed by 1999.
8. There are too many "fund-raisers" (cake sales without profits).

9. Visiting-hours policy should be enforced as far as hours and number of visitors (use role play and list of "polite enforcement techniques" as part of orientation and training).
10. Employee selection is naturally difficult due to the organization's location and limited supply of qualified candidates.

Issue 9: "From the List"

Considering the list of original recommendations and conclusions from the organizational study, the management group offered the following insights:

1. Mission awareness education and activity should be undertaken.
2. Part-time employees should be included in benefits (educate as to "why not").
3. Performance evaluation should be merit based (see issue 7).
4. Selection system should be uniform.
5. Training/education is needed in some areas on "union utopia"/"fact versus fiction" (for example, conduct "minisessions").
6. Discount should be enacted for each additional child utilizing the organization's day care center.
7. Educate employees on 1990s health care industry "facts of life" (use Delphi techniques).

Overall Conclusions and Recommendations

1. *Conclusion:* HMO coverage is desired by a number of employees.
   Recommendation: Explore and implement HMO business relations or explain organization's position to employees.
2. *Conclusion:* A significant number of employees are dissatisfied with the current benefits package.
   Recommendation: Review specific comments, weigh the level of dissatisfaction against collective perception, and either revamp aspects of the package or communicate the restraints that all businesses are under regarding benefits.
3. *Conclusion:* Salary levels are regarded as unfair among certain employees.
   Recommendation: Present a comprehensive wage survey to the employees and elicit their participation in the data collection process.
4. *Conclusion:* A variety of issues seem to be affecting the collective morale of the nursing department.
   Recommendation: Coordinate meetings with CEO, DON, and appropriate managers and staff members to discuss and address significant issues.

5. *Conclusion:* Marginal performance is perceived as being acceptable and in turn affects morale and productivity.
   Recommendation: Increase executive emphasis on documentation and performance assessment strategies.

6. *Conclusion:* Selection practices are not seen as optimally effective.
   Recommendation: Increase managerial and supervisory awareness and training in this area and consider implementing a structured selection system.

7. *Conclusion:* Certain employees perceive the construction project as a negative endeavor.
   Recommendation: Educate employees not only on need for the organization and its community, but also on the national issues mandating such projects.

8. *Conclusion:* A considerable amount of union sentiment exists in certain sectors of the organization's employee population.
   Recommendation: Conduct awareness education, particularly a "fact versus fiction" program.

9. *Conclusion:* Supervisory training is considered substandard.
   Recommendation: Implement a basic management modular training system.

10. *Conclusion:* The organization's "Future Vision" is unclear to some employees.
    Recommendation: Utilize the newsletter and other communication tools to give the employees a sense of future plans and objectives.

11. *Conclusion:* Morale seems to be enhanced by group activities.
    Recommendation: Build on programs like the employee picnic. Whenever appropriate, ask for employee input on such activities.

12. *Conclusion:* The organization's day care center is too small and too expensive.
    Recommendation: Explore expanding scope of the facility and fee structure for employees.

13. *Conclusion:* Pharmacy plan is cited as being limited and too expensive.
    Recommendation: Consider cost-effective methods of improving service and utilization of the plan (reduced cost, increased volume, and so on).

14. *Conclusion:* Overall survey results were quite positive across the board.
    Recommendation: Publish results throughout the organization as appropriate.

15. *Conclusion:* Many meetings are seen as being counterproductive.
    Recommendation: Conduct more efficient meeting-management training to include definitive objectives, scheduling techniques, and other management dynamics.

16. *Conclusion:* Customer satisfaction is perceived as positive, and the organization is a respected, valued community asset, as per feedback to employees in community.

Recommendation: Stress positive customer satisfaction perception to employees as motivational strategy and consider augmenting with community survey and marketing data collection.

17. *Conclusion:* Certain employees are not comfortable with the organization being so growth oriented and patients being customers.

    Recommendation: Emphasize the business reality of the current health care environment and link quality and "patient-first" ideals to good professional practices.

18. *Conclusion:* Positive physician relations are perceived by the majority of employees.

    Recommendation: Publicize the fact that the organization is unique in this regard, and consider specific dynamics that contribute to this situation.

19. *Conclusion:* Positive ethical action is perceived by the majority of employees.

    Recommendation: Maximize this perception through all aspects of value-driven management.

20. *Conclusion:* Survey comments have provided some specific "building blocks" for the organization's management.

    Recommendation: Set an incremental strategic plan to review progressive action quarterly.